Table of Contents

Secret Key #1 - Time is Your Greatest Enemy

Pace Yourself

Wear a watch. At the beginning of the test, check the time (or start a chronometer on your watch to count the minutes), and check the time after every few questions to make sure you are "on schedule."

If you are forced to speed up, do it efficiently. Usually one or more answer choices can be eliminated without too much difficulty. Above all, don't panic. Don't speed up and just begin guessing at random choices. By pacing yourself, and continually monitoring your progress against your watch, you will always know exactly how far ahead or behind you are with your available time. If you find that you are one minute behind on the test, don't skip one question without spending any time on it, just to catch back up. Take 15 fewer seconds on the next four questions, and after four questions you'll have caught back up. Once you catch back up, you can continue working each problem at your normal pace.

Furthermore, don't dwell on the problems that you were rushed on. If a problem was taking up too much time and you made a hurried guess, it must be difficult. The difficult questions are the ones you are most likely to miss anyway, so it isn't a big loss. It is better to end with more time than you need than to run out of time.

Lastly, sometimes it is beneficial to slow down if you are constantly getting ahead of time. You are always more likely to catch a careless mistake by working more slowly than quickly, and among very high-scoring test takers (those who are likely to have lots of time left over), careless errors affect the score more than mastery of material.

Secret Key #2 - Guessing is not Guesswork

You probably know that guessing is a good idea - unlike other standardized tests, there is no penalty for getting a wrong answer. Even if you have no idea about a question, you still have a 20-25% chance of getting it right.

Most test takers do not understand the impact that proper guessing can have on their score. Unless you score extremely high, guessing will significantly contribute to your final score.

Monkeys Take the Test

What most test takers don't realize is that to insure that 20-25% chance, you have to guess randomly. If you put 20 monkeys in a room to take this test, assuming they answered once per question and behaved themselves, on average they would get 20-25% of the questions correct. Put 20 test takers in the room, and the average will be much lower among guessed questions. Why?

1. The test writers intentionally write deceptive answer choices that "look" right. A test taker has no idea about a question, so picks the "best looking" answer, which is often wrong. The monkey has no idea what looks good and what doesn't, so will consistently be lucky about 20-25% of the time.
2. Test takers will eliminate answer choices from the guessing pool based on a hunch or intuition.

Simple but correct answers often get excluded, leaving a 0% chance of being correct. The monkey has no clue, and often gets lucky with the best choice.

This is why the process of elimination endorsed by most test courses is flawed and detrimental to your performance- test takers don't guess, they make an ignorant stab in the dark that is usually worse than random.

$5 Challenge

Let me introduce one of the most valuable ideas of this course- the $5 challenge:

You only mark your "best guess" if you are willing to bet $5 on it.
You only eliminate choices from guessing if you are willing to bet $5 on it.

Why $5? Five dollars is an amount of money that is small yet not insignificant, and can really add up fast (20 questions could cost you $100). Likewise, each answer choice on one question of the test will have a small impact on your overall score, but it can really add up to a lot of points in the end.

The process of elimination IS valuable. The following shows your chance of guessing it right:

If you eliminate wrong answer choices until only this many remain:	Chance of getting it correct:
1	100%
2	50%
3	33%

However, if you accidentally eliminate the right answer or go on a hunch for an incorrect answer, your chances drop dramatically: to 0%. By guessing among all the answer choices, you are

GUARANTEED to have a shot at the right answer.

That's why the $5 test is so valuable- if you give up the advantage and safety of a pure guess, it had better be worth the risk.

What we still haven't covered is how to be sure that whatever guess you make is truly random. Here's the easiest way:

Always pick the first answer choice among those remaining.

Such a technique means that you have decided, **before you see a single test question**, exactly how you are going to guess- and since the order of choices tells you nothing about which one is correct, this guessing technique is perfectly random.

This section is not meant to scare you away from making educated guesses or eliminating choices- you just need to define when a choice is worth eliminating. The $5 test, along with a pre-defined random guessing strategy, is the best way to make sure you reap all of the benefits of guessing.

Secret Key #3 - Practice Smarter, Not Harder

Many test takers delay the test preparation process because they dread the awful amounts of practice time they think necessary to succeed on the test. We have refined an effective method that will take you only a fraction of the time.

There are a number of "obstacles" in your way to succeed. Among these are answering questions, finishing in time, and mastering test-taking strategies. All must be executed on the day of the test at peak performance, or your score will suffer. The test is a mental marathon that has a large impact on your future.

Just like a marathon runner, it is important to work your way up to the full challenge. So first you just worry about questions, and then time, and finally strategy:

Success Strategy

1. Find a good source for practice tests.
2. If you are willing to make a larger time investment, consider using more than one study guide- often the different approaches of multiple authors will help you "get" difficult concepts.
3. Take a practice test with no time constraints, with all study helps "open book." Take your time with questions and focus on applying strategies.
4. Take a practice test with time constraints, with all guides "open book."
5. Take a final practice test with no open material and time limits

If you have time to take more practice tests, just repeat step 5. By gradually exposing yourself to the full rigors of the test environment, you will condition your mind to the stress of test day and maximize your success.

Secret Key #4 - Prepare, Don't Procrastinate

Let me state an obvious fact: if you take the test three times, you will get three different scores. This is due to the way you feel on test day, the level of preparedness you have, and, despite the test writers' claims to the contrary, some tests WILL be easier for you than others.

Since your future depends so much on your score, you should maximize your chances of success. In order to maximize the likelihood of success, you've got to prepare in advance. This means taking practice tests and spending time learning the information and test taking strategies you will need to succeed.
Never take the test as a "practice" test, expecting that you can just take it again if you need to. Feel free to take sample tests on your own, but when you go to take the official test, be prepared, be focused, and do your best the first time!

Secret Key #5 - Test Yourself

Everyone knows that time is money. There is no need to spend too much of your time or too little of your time preparing for the test. You should only spend as much of your precious time preparing as is necessary for you to get the score you need.

Once you have taken a practice test under real conditions of time constraints, then you will know if you are ready for the test or not.
If you have scored extremely high the first

time that you take the practice test, then there is not much point in spending countless hours studying. You are already there.

Benchmark your abilities by retaking practice tests and seeing how much you have improved. Once you score high enough to guarantee success, then you are ready.

If you have scored well below where you need, then knuckle down and begin studying in earnest. Check your improvement regularly through the use of practice tests under real conditions. Above all, don't worry, panic, or give up. The key is perseverance!

Then, when you go to take the test, remain confident and remember how well you did on the practice tests. If you can score high enough on a practice test, then you can do the same on the real thing.

General Strategies

The most important thing you can do is to ignore your fears and jump into the test immediately- do not be overwhelmed by any strange-sounding terms. You have to jump into the test like jumping into a pool- all at once is the easiest way.

Make Predictions

As you read and understand the question, try to guess what the answer will be. Remember that several of the answer choices are wrong, and once you begin reading them, your mind will immediately become cluttered with answer choices designed to throw you off. Your mind is typically the most focused immediately after you have read the question and digested its contents. If you can, try to predict what the correct answer will be.

You may be surprised at what you can predict.

Quickly scan the choices and see if your prediction is in the listed answer choices. If it is, then you can be quite confident that you have the right answer. It still won't hurt to check the other answer choices, but most of the time, you've got it!

Answer the Question

It may seem obvious to only pick answer choices that answer the question, but the test writers can create some excellent answer choices that are wrong. Don't pick an answer just because it sounds right, or you believe it to be true. It MUST answer the question. Once you've made your selection, always go back and check it against the question and make sure that you didn't misread the question, and the answer choice does answer the question posed.

Benchmark

After you read the first answer choice, decide if you think it sounds correct or not. If it doesn't, move on to the next answer choice. If it does, mentally mark that answer choice. This doesn't mean that you've definitely selected it as your answer choice, it just means that it's the best you've seen thus far. Go ahead and read the next choice. If the next choice is worse than the one you've already selected, keep going to the next answer choice. If the next choice is better than the choice you've already selected, mentally mark the new answer choice as your best guess.

The first answer choice that you select becomes your standard. Every other answer choice must be benchmarked against that standard. That choice is correct until proven otherwise by another answer choice beating it out. Once you've decided that no other answer choice seems as good, do one final check to ensure that your answer choice answers the question posed.

Valid Information

Don't discount any of the information provided in the question. Every piece of information may be necessary to determine the correct answer. None of the information in the question is there to throw you off (while the answer choices will certainly have information to throw you off). If two seemingly unrelated topics are discussed, don't ignore either. You can be confident there is a relationship, or it wouldn't be included in the question, and you are probably going to have to determine what is that relationship to find the answer.

Avoid "Fact Traps"

Don't get distracted by a choice that is factually true. Your search is for the answer that answers the question. Stay focused and don't fall for an answer that is true but incorrect. Always go back to the question and make sure you're choosing an answer that actually answers the question and is not just a true statement. An answer can be factually correct, but it MUST answer the question asked. Additionally, two answers can both be seemingly correct, so be sure to read all of the answer choices, and make sure that you get the one that BEST answers the question.

Milk the Question

Some of the questions may throw you completely off. They might deal with a subject you have not been exposed to, or one that you haven't reviewed in years. While your lack of knowledge about the subject will be a hindrance, the question itself can give you many clues that will help you find the correct answer. Read the question carefully and look for clues. Watch particularly for adjectives and nouns describing difficult terms or words

that you don't recognize. Regardless of if you completely understand a word or not, replacing it with a synonym either provided or one you more familiar with may help you to understand what the questions are asking. Rather than wracking your mind about specific detailed information concerning a difficult term or word, try to use mental substitutes that are easier to understand.

The Trap of Familiarity

Don't just choose a word because you recognize it. On difficult questions, you may not recognize a number of words in the answer choices. The test writers don't put "make-believe" words on the test; so don't think that just because you only recognize all the words in one answer choice means that answer choice must be correct. If you only recognize words in one answer choice, then focus on that one. Is it correct? Try your best to determine if it is correct. If it is, that is great, but if it doesn't, eliminate it. Each word and answer choice you eliminate increases your chances of getting the question correct, even if you then have to guess among the unfamiliar choices.

Eliminate Answers

Eliminate choices as soon as you realize they are wrong. But be careful! Make sure you consider all of the possible answer choices. Just because one appears right, doesn't mean that the next one won't be even better! The test writers will usually put more than one good answer choice for every question, so read all of them. Don't worry if you are stuck between two that seem right. By getting down to just two remaining possible choices, your odds are now 50/50. Rather than wasting too much time, play the odds. You are guessing, but guessing wisely, because you've been able to knock out some of the answer choices that you know are wrong. If you are eliminating choices and realize that the last answer choice you are left with is also obviously wrong, don't panic. Start over and consider each choice again. There may easily be something that you missed the first time and will realize on the second pass.

Tough Questions

If you are stumped on a problem or it appears too hard or too difficult, don't waste time. Move on! Remember though, if you can quickly check for obviously incorrect answer choices, your chances of guessing correctly are greatly improved. Before you completely give up, at least try to knock out a couple of possible answers. Eliminate what you can and then guess at the remaining answer choices before moving on.

Brainstorm

If you get stuck on a difficult question, spend a few seconds quickly brainstorming. Run through the complete list of possible answer choices. Look at each choice and ask yourself, "Could this answer the question satisfactorily?" Go through each answer choice and consider it independently of the other. By systematically going through all possibilities, you may find something that you would otherwise overlook. Remember that when you get stuck, it's important to try to keep moving.

Read Carefully

Understand the problem. Read the question and answer choices carefully. Don't miss the question because you misread the terms. You have plenty of time to read each question thoroughly and make sure you understand what is being asked. Yet a happy medium must be attained, so don't waste too much time. You must read carefully, but efficiently.

Face Value

When in doubt, use common sense. Always accept the situation in the problem at face value. Don't read too much into it. These problems will not require you to make huge leaps of logic. The test writers aren't trying to throw you off with a cheap trick. If you have to go beyond creativity and make a leap of logic in order to have an answer choice answer the question, then you should look at the other answer choices. Don't overcomplicate the problem by creating theoretical relationships or explanations that will warp time or space. These are normal problems rooted in reality. It's just that the applicable relationship or explanation may not be readily apparent and you have to figure things out. Use your common sense to interpret anything that isn't clear.

Prefixes

If you're having trouble with a word in the question or answer choices, try dissecting it. Take advantage of every clue that the word might include. Prefixes and suffixes can be a huge help. Usually they allow you to determine a basic meaning. Pre- means before, post- means after, pro - is positive, de- is negative. From these prefixes and suffixes, you can get an idea of the general meaning of the word and try to put it into context. Beware though of any traps. Just because con is the opposite of pro, doesn't necessarily mean congress is the opposite of progress!

Hedge Phrases

Watch out for critical "hedge" phrases, such as likely, may, can, will often, sometimes, often, almost, mostly, usually, generally, rarely, sometimes. Question writers insert these hedge phrases to cover every possibility. Often an answer choice will be wrong simply because it leaves no room for exception. Avoid answer choices that have definitive words like "exactly," and "always".

Switchback Words

Stay alert for "switchbacks". These are the words and phrases frequently used to alert you to shifts in thought. The most common switchback word is "but". Others include although, however, nevertheless, on the other hand, even though, while, in spite of, despite, regardless of.

New Information

Correct answer choices will rarely have completely new information included. Answer choices typically are straightforward reflections of the material asked about and will directly relate to the question. If a new piece of information is included in an answer choice that doesn't even seem to relate to the topic being asked about, then that answer choice is likely incorrect. All of the information needed to answer the question is usually provided for you, and so you should not have to make guesses that are unsupported or choose answer choices that require unknown information that cannot be reasoned on its own.

Time Management

On technical questions, don't get lost on the technical terms. Don't spend too much time on any one question. If you don't know what a term means, then since you don't have a dictionary, odds are you aren't going to get much further. You should immediately recognize terms as whether or not you know them. If you don't, work with the other clues that you have, the other answer choices and terms provided, but don't waste too much time trying to figure out a difficult term.

Contextual Clues

Look for contextual clues. An answer can be right but not correct. The contextual clues will help you find the answer that is most right and is correct. Understand the context in which a phrase or statement is made. This will help you make important distinctions.

Don't Panic

Panicking will not answer any questions for you. Therefore, it isn't helpful. When you first see the question, if your mind goes blank, take a deep breath. Force yourself to mechanically go through the steps of solving the problem and using the strategies you've learned.

Pace Yourself

Don't get clock fever. It's easy to be overwhelmed when you're looking at a page full of questions, your mind is full of random thoughts and feeling confused, and the clock is ticking down faster than you would like. Calm down and maintain the pace that you have set for yourself. As long as you are on track by monitoring your pace, you are guaranteed to have enough time for yourself. When you get to the last few minutes of the test, it may seem like you won't have enough time left, but if you only have as many questions as you should have left at that point, then you're right on track!

Answer Selection

The best way to pick an answer choice is to eliminate all of those that are wrong, until only one is left and confirm that is the correct answer. Sometimes though, an answer choice may immediately look right. Be careful! Take a second to make sure that the other choices are not equally obvious. Don't make a hasty mistake. There are only two times that you should stop before checking other answers. First is when you are positive that the answer choice you have selected is correct. Second is when time is almost out and you have to make a quick guess!

Check Your Work

Since you will probably not know every term listed and the answer to every question, it is important that you get credit for the ones that you do know. Don't miss any questions through careless mistakes. If at all possible, try to take a second to look back over your answer selection and make sure you've selected the correct answer choice and haven't made a costly careless mistake (such as marking an answer choice that you didn't mean to mark). This quick double check should more than pay for itself in caught mistakes for the time it costs.

Beware of Directly Quoted Answers

Sometimes an answer choice will repeat word for word a portion of the question or reference section. However, beware of such exact duplication – it may be a trap! More than likely, the correct choice will paraphrase or summarize a point, rather than being exactly the same wording.

Slang

Scientific sounding answers are better than slang ones. An answer choice that begins "To compare the outcomes…" is much more likely to be correct than one that begins "Because some people insisted…"

Extreme Statements

s a radical iAvoid wild answers that throw out highly controversial ideas that are proclaimed as established fact. An answer choice that states the "process should used in certain situations, if…" is much more likely to be correct than one that states the "process should be discontinued completely." The first is a calm rational statement and doesn't even make a definitive, uncompromising stance, using a hedge word "if" to provide wiggle room, whereas the second choice idea and far more extreme.

Answer Choice Families

When you have two or more answer choices that are direct opposites or parallels, one of them is usually the correct answer. For instance, if one answer choice states "x increases" and another answer choice states "x decreases" or "y increases," then those two or three answer choices are very similar in construction and fall into the same family of answer choices. A family of answer choices is when two or three answer choices are very similar in construction, and yet often have a directly opposite meaning. Usually the correct answer choice will be in that family of answer choices. The "odd man out" or answer choice that doesn't seem to fit the parallel construction of the other answer choices is more likely to be incorrect.

Top 20 Test Taking Tips

1. Carefully follow all the test registration procedures
2. Know the test directions, duration, topics, question types, how many questions
3. Setup a flexible study schedule at least 3-4 weeks before test day
4. Study during the time of day you are most alert, relaxed, and stress free
5. Maximize your learning style; visual learner use visual study aids, auditory learner use auditory study aids
6. Focus on your weakest knowledge base
7. Find a study partner to review with and help clarify questions
8. Practice, practice, practice
9. Get a good night's sleep; don't try to cram the night before the test
10. Eat a well balanced meal
11. Know the exact physical location of the testing site; drive the route to the site prior to test day
12. Bring a set of ear plugs; the testing center could be noisy
13. Wear comfortable, loose fitting, layered clothing to the testing center; prepare for it to be either cold or hot during the test
14. Bring at least 2 current forms of ID to the testing center
15. Arrive to the test early; be prepared to wait and be patient
16. Eliminate the obviously wrong answer choices, then guess the first remaining choice
17. Pace yourself; don't rush, but keep working and move on if you get stuck
18. Maintain a positive attitude even if the test is going poorly
19. Keep your first answer unless you are positive it is wrong
20. Check your work, don't make a careless mistake

ARRT Nuclear Medicine Technology

Radiation Protection

Direct and indirect action

Direct action refers to cellular damage in response to direct absorption of ionizing radiation. This type of ionization occurs at all levels of radiation; the greater the exposure to radiation, the greater the amount of cellular damage.

Indirect action refers to the production of a free radical as a result of radiation exposure. A free radical is an electrically neutral atom with an unoccupied electron. Since the primary atom in the body is water, radiation exposure can break water down into a hydrogen atom (H+) and a hydroxide ion (OH-). When many of these hydroxide ion free radicals are present in the body, the formation of toxic hydrogen peroxide (H_2O_2) may result.

RBE

Relative Biologic Effectiveness refers to the fact that different types of radiation produce different biologic effects. RBE primarily is the ratio of an absorbed dose of x-rays or gamma rays to the amount of any other form of radiation that is needed to produce the same biologic effect. RBE is calculated by the following formula:

$$RBE = \frac{Dose\ of\ x-ray\ or\ gamma\ radiation}{Equivalent\ dose\ of\ radiation\ in\ question}$$

For example, if 0.05 rad of alpha radiation produces the same effect as 1 rad of gamma radiation, the RBE for alpha radiation would be the following:

$$RBE = \frac{1\ rad}{0.05\ rad} = 20$$

Stochastic effects of radiation

Stochastic effects of radiation are generally associated with exposure to low-level radiation over a prolonged period of time. Long-term exposure to low-level radiation can lead to leukemia and other forms of cancer. This type of radiation exposure can also alter human genetics—causing chromosome damage, for example—due to its effects at the cellular level. Genetic effects of this kind are difficult to quantify, however. Long-term, low-level radiation exposure has been associated with genetic birth defects, too, but it is extremely difficult to determine what percentages of those are related to radiation exposure.

Deterministic effects of radiation

Deterministic effects of radiation can also be referred to as non-stochastic radiation effects. Deterministic effects are a result of a high dose of radiation over a short period of time. These types of effects are directly proportional to the amount of radiation exposure; the greater the amount of radiation exposure, the more severe the biological effect. Deterministic effects can vary from redness of the skin to death in some cases. Depending on the dose of radiation absorbed, deterministic events can be immediate, as with very high levels of radiation, or may take a few days to develop, as might occur with relatively low levels of radiation.

ALARA

ALARA stands for As Low As Reasonably Achievable. This principle is aimed at reducing radiation exposure in individuals who work routinely with radiation. ALARA is achieved by using protective equipment such as syringe shields, lead glass and lead shields. Reducing contact time with and maintaining distance from radioactive sources, including patients in a nuclear medicine setting, will also help keep radiation exposure as low as reasonably achievable.

Distance from radioactive sources

Maintaining distance from a radioactive source is one of the most effective and least expensive ways to reduce radiation exposure. The "*inverse square law*" tells us that if the distance from a radioactive source is doubled, the radiation exposure is one-fourth of that at the original distance. Conversely, if the distance from a radioactive source is halved, the radiation exposure is 4 times greater than at the original distance.

Radiation exposure measurements

There are three basic measures of radiation exposure—roentgen (R), radiation absorbed dose (rad), and radiation equivalent to man (rem). Roentgen, a term applied to x-rays and gamma rays, is the amount of radiation it takes to produce 1 electrostatic charge in 1cc of dry air at standard temperature and pressure. Rad differs from roentgen in that it encompasses all types of radiation, not just x-rays and gamma rays. In addition, rad can be measured in types of matter other than air. Rem is the unit of measure applied to radiation exposure in humans. It is calculated by multiplying the number of rads by the relative biologic effectiveness (RBE).

Radiation exposure regulations

The Nuclear Regulatory Commission (NRC) has established annual radiation exposure limits for humans. These limits can vary for different segments of the population. A member of the general public should be exposed to no greater than 100 millirem (mrem) per year. Individuals who are radiation workers can be exposed to a maximum of 5,000 mrem per year unless they are minors, in which case the annual maximum is 500 mrem. A female radiation worker who declares a pregnancy may only be exposed to 500 mrem throughout her nine-month pregnancy. Radiation workers may have certain body parts monitored. The maximum permissible radiation dose to the eye, for example, is 15,000 mrem per year. The skin and extremities should be exposed to no more than 50,000 mrem per year.

Personnel monitoring devices

According to NRC regulations, all film badges should be worn in the area of the body at risk of greatest radiation exposure, usually the chest or collar area. Under no circumstances should a monitoring device be worn under a lead apron. Individuals who wear devices on fingers, such as nuclear medicine technologists, should not have the device facing away from the palm. Finger badges should be worn so they are facing the radioactive material while an injection is being performed.

NRC reportable events

According to the NRC, there are three events that must be reported: the administration of therapeutic radiation doses, such as I-131, to the wrong patient, an administered dose that exceeds 20% of the total prescribed dose, and a single therapeutic dose that varies by more than

20% from the written directive or a weekly therapeutic dose that varies by more than 30% from the written directive.

Radiation contamination check

An area survey using a Geiger counter should be performed daily to check for radioactive contamination in areas where radiopharmaceuticals are assayed, prepared, and administered. The stress testing/treadmill area should be part of a daily survey. An area survey should be performed on a weekly basis in all areas where radiopharmaceuticals are stored and where radioactive waste is placed for decay. In addition, a wipe test should be performed on a weekly basis in all areas where radioactive materials are prepared, administered, or stored. Each wipe must encompass an area of at least 100 square centimeters.

Contaminated area classification

Contaminated areas are classified by the type of area being surveyed and the type of isotope an area is contaminated with. Restricted areas are areas such as the hot lab and stress testing area where radioactive materials are routinely prepared and administered. A restricted area is considered to be contaminated if a wipe test delivers a result greater than 20,000 DPM/100 cm^2 for isotopes such as Tc-99m or Tl-201. The threshold for a restricted area is lowered to 2,000 DPM/100 cm^2 if the area is contaminated with a high-energy isotope such as I-131 or In-111.

Warning signs of radioactivity

Several types of warning signs are posted in medical settings. These signs must accurately identify the type of radiation that may be encountered. A "*Caution Radioactive Materials*" sign posted 30 cm from the radiation source is sufficient for areas with a radiation level below 5 mR/hr. A "*Caution Radiation Area*" sign must be posted 30 cm from the radiation source or radioactive surface in all areas that have a radiation level greater than 5 mR/hr. A "*Caution High Radiation Area*" sign is required in all areas in which the radiation level exceeds 100 mR/hr. This, too, should be posted 30 cm from the radiation source or radioactive surface.

Decontamination of a radioactive spill

Typically, the person responsible for a radioactive spill is responsible for the decontamination efforts. The first thing to do is assess the spill for amount of radiation, type of isotope, and extent of contamination. Second, the spill should be contained to prevent contamination of other areas. Third, the contaminated area should be made off limits to all persons not involved with decontamination procedures. The contaminated area should be clearly marked by signs or other easily noticed warnings. Decontamination efforts should continue until the wipe test of the area is below 200 DPM/cm^2.

Radioactive packages labeling

There are several different shipping labels for radioactive packages. A radioactive package should have a White I label if the package has a surface radiation level less than 0.5 mR/hr and a 0 transportation index at 1 meter. A Yellow II label is required if a radioactive package has a surface radiation level greater than 0.5 mR/hr but less than 50 mR/hr and a transport index greater than 0 but less than 1.0 at 1 meter. A Yellow III label is used on packages with surface radiation levels greater than 50 mR/hr but less than 200 mR/hr and transport indexes greater than 1 but less than 10 at 1 meter. A Yellow III Exclusive Use label is used on all packages with surface radiation levels greater than 200 mR/hr but less than 1,000 mR/hr and transport indexes greater than 10 at 1 meter.

Radioactive waste disposal

Several different methods may be used to legally dispose of radioactive waste. Radioactive patient excreta such as urine and feces can be legally disposed of by releasing them into the sanitary sewage systems. The most common form of disposal is simply to store the waste until the radiation levels decay to background level, then dispose of the waste in regular trash or biohazard trash. In addition, the waste can be transferred to an authorized recipient for disposal. When this method is selected, the waste must be in the proper container with the proper shipping labels in order to transport it legally.

Sealed radioactive sources
Sealed radioactive sources should be stored in a very specific manner. Each sealed source should have its own individual container so it cannot become lost and to make inventory easier. To ensure proper accountability of sealed sources, they should be inventoried at least quarterly during a formal audit of the nuclear medicine facility. In addition, if any new sealed sources are acquired between audits, the new sources should be added to the inventory upon receipt.

Decayed in storage

Radioactive waste can legally be decayed in storage if the isotopes contained in the waste have a physical half-life of less than 65 days. In addition, the radioactive waste must be held in storage for no less than 10 half-lives and must emit no measurable radiation. If the waste is held for 10 half-lives and radiation is detected from the waste, it needs to be held for a longer period until no radiation can be detected.

Radionuclide's and radiopharmaceuticals

Radioactive decay

Radioactive decay is the manner in which an unstable atomic nucleus loses energy by producing ionizing particles in an effort to become stable. In any method of radioactive decay, the original unstable atom is known as the parent, and the atom it decays into is known as the daughter. If the daughter atom is stable, the radioactive decay process is complete. If the daughter atom is still unstable, the radioactive decay process continues until a stable atom is achieved.

Alpha decay

Alpha decay is a radioactive decay process in which the unstable atom emits an alpha particle in order to achieve stability. An alpha particle has an atomic structure identical to a helium atom—2 protons and 2 neutrons. Alpha particles are denoted by the Greek symbol α or the chemical formula for Helium nuclei, which is ^4_2He. Alpha decay typically occurs in heavier atoms such as uranium-238 and the daughter atom is lighter than the parent atom by the amount of a helium atom. The decay of uranium-238 results in the daughter atom thorium-234 and an alpha particle. The alpha decay structure of uranium-238 is documented with the following decay equation:

$$^{238}_{92}U \rightarrow\ ^{234}_{90}Th + ^4_2He$$

Beta decay

Beta decay is a radioactive decay process in which an unstable atom emits a beta particle in order to achieve stability. This form of decay can result in 2 different particles being emitted, either an electron or a positron. If an electron is emitted, the particle is referred to as a beta minus (β^-). If a positron is emitted, the particle is referred to as a beta plus (β^+). In beta minus decay, the atomic number of the daughter atom increases by 1. In beta plus decay, the atomic number of the daughter atom decreases by 1.

Gamma decay

Gamma decay is unlike alpha, beta minus, or beta plus decay in that the atomic number of the parent and daughter atoms are identical. In alpha or beta decay, an atom is frequently left in an excited state. In order for the nucleus to remove itself from the excited state and return to the stable, ground state, it must emit energy. The energy emitted from these nuclei is in the form of photons referred to as gamma rays. For isotopes that use gamma decay, all photons that are emitted contain the same energy and ionization properties.

Bremsstrahlung

Bremsstrahlung is the production of electromagnetic radiation caused by the sudden deceleration or deflection of a fast-moving charged particle when it collides with another charged particle. This phenomenon occurs primarily when beta particles pass near an atomic nucleus. The beta particles and atomic nucleus are attracted to each other due to opposite electrical charges. The beta particles change direction, slow down and move toward the atomic nucleus. The slowing of the beta particles causes a reduction of kinetic energy within the particles. The kinetic energy is lost in the form of x-rays. The energy of the x-rays is equal to the amount of kinetic energy lost by the beta particles.

Compton scatter

Compton scatter occurs when a gamma ray interacts with a free or loosely bound electron. During this interaction, some of the energy from the gamma ray is absorbed into the electron. The amount of energy absorbed depends on the angle of interaction between the gamma ray and electron. If they collide head on, the majority of the gamma rays energy will be transferred to the electron. If the collision occurs at different angles, a lesser amount of energy will be transferred from the gamma ray to the electron. Compton scatter removes the electron from its orbit and results in a reduced-energy gamma ray.

Photoelectric effect

The photoelectric effect occurs when a gamma ray interacts with an electron on an inner orbit. During this interaction, the energy from the gamma ray is totally absorbed by the inner-orbit electron. The electron that absorbs the gamma ray is referred to as a photoelectron. The photoelectron is ejected from its orbit and the atom. The energy of the photoelectron is equal to the energy of the gamma ray minus the binding energy the electron needed to remain in its orbits. Due to the vacancy of an inner-orbit electron, outer-orbit electrons will drop down to fill the space left by the photoelectron and a series of x-rays will be emitted for every electron that changes orbit.

Pair production

Pair production occurs when a gamma ray reaches the vicinity of a nucleus. The energy of the gamma ray is totally absorbed by the electrical field of the nucleus, thus yielding the production of a beta particle and a positron. Pair production will only occur if the gamma ray has a minimum energy of 1.022 MeV.

The beta particle travels until it is incorporated into an atom or acts as a free electron. The positron inevitably collides with an electron, resulting in annihilation of both particles and the emission of 2 gamma rays with 511 keV of energy.

Auger electrons

Auger electrons are produced when an inner-shell electron is released from its orbit, leaving a vacancy. When there is a vacancy on an inner shell, outer-shell electrons adjust and move closer to the core, filling the vacancy. Every time an electron moves to a different shell, energy is released. Sometimes the energy is released in the form of a photon. Other times, the energy is transferred to an outer-shell electron, which is then released from the atom. An Auger electron is one that absorbs the energy and is subsequently released from the atom.

Physical half-life

Physical half-life, also referred to as radioactive half-life, is the amount of time it takes for the original number of atoms in a radioactive sample to be reduced by 50%. This may also be referred to as radioactive decay and is a characteristic of all radioactive materials. Each radioactive isotope has a different rate of decay or half-life. However, the rate of decay for each radioisotope in constant and cannot be altered by outside influences such as temperature or pressure.

Biological half-life

Biological half-life is defined as the amount of time it takes the body to eliminate half the quantity of any substance, not just radioactivity. Biological half-life is the same for both stable and radioactive forms of any element. The body's main methods of eliminating substances are genitourinary excretion, gastrointestinal excretion, exhalation, and perspiration.

Effective half-life

Effective half-life is defined as the amount of time required to reduce the quantity of a substance in the body when both physical and biological half-life are taken into consideration. Effective half-life combines the action of radioactive decay and natural elimination. Effective half-life can be calculated in the following equation:

$$\frac{1}{t_{eff}} = \frac{1}{t_{biol}} + \frac{1}{t_{phys}}$$

Capillary blockade

The mode of uptake known as capillary blockade occurs when radioactive particles are injected intravenously into a patient, and the radioactive particles become trapped in the capillary beds of the patient. This mode of uptake is primarily associated with pulmonary perfusion imaging in which Tc-99m MAA is injected intravenously and the Tc-99m MAA particles become trapped in the capillaries of the lungs. The average adult capillary measures 7 mm in diameter. Tc-99m MAA particles must have sizes ranging from 10 mm to 90 mm, thus allowing for capillary blockade in the lungs.

Active transport

Active transport is defined as the utilization of a normal metabolic pathway to allow the radiopharmaceutical to penetrate the cell membrane and incorporate itself into the cell. Thyroid imaging is possible because iodine is incorporated into the thyroid via active transport. Iodine becomes trapped in the thyroid and is converted into T3 and T4. Cardiac imaging with thallium or rubidium uses active transport as a method of localization in the heart. Thallium and rubidium are potassium analogs and therefore use the sodium/potassium pump mechanism to incorporate into the heart.

Phagocytosis

Phagocytosis is defined as the engulfment of solid particles by cells known as phagocytes. Kupffer cells which are located in the liver act as phagocytes for uptake of radioactive particles. Intravenous injection of Tc-99m sulfur colloid is localized in the liver due to phagocytosis. In order for this to occur, the average particle size for Tc-99m sulfur colloid must be between 0.1 and 2.0 μm since the average capillary size in the liver is 7 μm. Particle size is extremely important for Tc-99m sulfur colloid to prevent capillary blockade from occurring.

Compartmental localization

Compartmental localization involves placing a radiopharmaceutical in a space and maintaining it in that space long enough to perform imaging. An example of this is pulmonary ventilation imaging, which is performed via inhalation of Tc-99m DTPA or Xe-133 gas directly into the lungs. MUGA scans also use compartmental localization. Imaging can be performed after Tc-99m-labeled red blood cells are injected intravenously into the blood. Cisternograms use compartmental localization, too, via In-111 DTPA administration directly into the cerebral spinal fluid by lumbar puncture.

Chemisorption

Chemisorption is defined as the chemical binding of a radiopharmaceutical to the surface of another substance. Skeletal imaging is obtained using chemisorption when Tc-99m MDP is injected intravenously and binds to the hydroxyapatite crystals of the bone. Acute myocardial infarction imaging is also performed using this process. When cardiac cells begin to die as a result of a myocardial infarction, some of the ions in the heart are converted to hydroxyapatite crystals. Tc-99m PYP, which is a phosphate similar to MDP, binds to the hydroxyapatite crystals so infarction imaging can be obtained. Imaging for acute venous thrombosis is made possible by chemisorption, too. Tc-99m AcuTect binds to the surface of the thrombus, enabling the thrombus to be imaged.

Oxidation/reduction reaction

Tc-99m needs to be in a reduced oxidation state in order to bind efficiently with the radiopharmaceutical. Most radiopharmaceuticals require the stannous (tin) ion in order to reduce the Tc-99m. If the compounded radiopharmaceutical is exposed to oxygen, the compound may have impurities. Most radiopharmaceuticals have more stannous ion than required to protect against oxidation. If oxidation occurs, the compound NaTcO4 may result. In addition, a hydrolyzed form of technetium that acts as a colloid may result. If the compound becomes hydrolyzed, liver uptake may be visible on skeletal imaging due to the technetium acting as a colloid.

Mo-99/Tc-99m breakthrough test

Mo-99 is the parent molecule of Tc-99m. The current regulations state that every time a Mo-99 generator is eluted, the Mo-

99/Tc-99m breakthrough test must be performed to evaluate the purity of Tc-99m. The Tc-99m that is eluted must not contain greater than 0.15 µCi of Mo-99 per 1 mCi of Tc-99m. If it does, the Tc-99m is deemed to be impure and should not be administered to patients.

Radiopharmaceutical kit preparation

In order to be in compliance with NRC regulations, every radiopharmaceutical that is compounded must be properly documented. For each radioactive kit that is prepared, the date and time of preparation, the lot number of the pharmaceutical, the expiration date of the pharmaceutical, the activity of the preparation (usually in mCi), the volume of the preparation (usually in mL), and the concentration of the preparation (usually in mCi/mL) must be documented to be in compliance with NRC regulations.

Whole-body skeletal imaging

Whole-body skeletal imaging is routinely performed for high-risk patients with malignant tumors that are known to metastasize to the bones. Tumors located in the breast, lung, and prostate are the most frequent primary cancers in which skeletal imaging is useful. Whole-body imaging is frequently performed following an elevated alkaline phosphatase blood result and as routine follow-up to therapeutic regimens such as radiation therapy and chemotherapy. Whole-body imaging may also be performed for persistent bone pain that is unexplained by other imaging modalities such as x-ray, CT scan, or MRI.

Procedure
Once the patient has completed the 3-hour waiting period following intravenous administration of Tc-99m MDP, the skeletal image can be acquired. Immediately prior to skeletal imaging, the patient is asked to void completely. This allows the contents of the bladder to be eliminated and the bone of the pelvis to be evaluated more clearly. To begin whole body imaging, instruct the patient to lie in a supine position on the imaging table. Make every effort to center the patient on the table to ensure the entire body will be imaged. Using a low-energy, high-resolution collimator, adjust the detector so it is as close to the patient as possible without touching him or her. Set the scan speed of the gamma camera to approximately 12 sec/cm. This scan speed will acquire the whole body image in approximately 20 minutes.

Three-phase skeletal imaging

Three-phase skeletal imaging is routinely performed in an attempt to diagnose osteomyelitis. This technique is also used for early detection of avascular necrosis. Three-phase bone scanning is particularly useful when attempting to diagnose a stress fracture or any occult skeletal trauma that may not be evident with other imaging modalities such as x-ray, CT scan, or MRI. In addition, three-phase bone imaging may be performed to evaluate soft tissue abnormalities such as cellulitis in order to detect any bone involvement that may be present with this condition.

Procedure
Prior to administration of Tc-99m MDP, the patient should be positioned under the gamma camera with the affected area positioned in the field of view. The flow phase of the acquisition should be obtained via dynamic imaging for a minimum of 10 frames at 5 seconds per frame. Immediately following the flow phase, the blood-pool image(s) should be acquired for approximately 500K counts. At this point, the 3-hour waiting period is begun to allow proper absorption of Tc-99m MDP into the bones. Once the 3-hour

waiting period is complete, delayed imaging is performed at similar parameters as the blood-pool phase to complete the third phase of the procedure.

Patient preparation
There is virtually no patient preparation for skeletal imaging prior to injection of Tc-99m MDP. Once the Tc-99m MDP has been administered, the patient must wait approximately 3 hours in order to allow for proper absorption of the radioisotope into the bones. Throughout the 3-hour waiting time, the patient is instructed to drink plenty of fluids. The added hydration will allow the Tc-99m MDP to wash out of the soft tissues of the body and enable the bones to be evaluated more clearly. In addition, the hydration and subsequent voiding will allow the patient to eliminate the Tc-99m MDP from the system more rapidly, thus reducing radiation exposure from the radioisotope. Once the 3-hour waiting time has elapsed and immediately prior to imaging, the patient is asked to void in order to evaluate the bones of the pelvis more clearly by eliminating the contents of the bladder.

Skeletal SPECT imaging

For nuclear medicine departments that routinely perform SPECT imaging, additional quality control measures should be taken in order to ensure technically adequate SPECT images. A center or rotation evaluation should be performed on a weekly basis. A bar-phantom image and, in some cases, a tomographic phantom image, should be acquired on a monthly basis. In order to perform the procedure, the gamma camera should be equipped with a low-energy, high-resolution collimator. The detectors should be programmed for a 360-degree rotation as close to the patient as possible. The SPECT images

should be acquired using a 128 x 128 matrix. The acquisition should be set for 64 frames at a minimum of 20 seconds per frame.

Tc-99m MDP

Tc-99m methyl diphosphonate is the radiopharmaceutical most commonly chosen for skeletal imaging. Tc-99m MDP is administered to the patient via intravenous injection. For skeletal imaging, Tc-99m MDP is administered in the activity range of 20 to 30 mCi. Tc-99m MDP is localized in the bones via chemisorption. Chemisorption is the process in which the radiotracer, Tc-99m MDP, becomes chemically bound to the hydroxyapatite structures of the bones.

Brain death study

Brain death studies are used to confirm brain death in patients who present with unresponsive coma, fixed and dilated pupils, and silent electroencephalogram. The procedure is performed by intravenous injection of Tc-99m pertechnetate, Tc-99m DTPA, or Tc-99m bicisate. A dynamic flow study is done initially for approximately 90 seconds at a rate of 2 seconds/frame. Approximately 15 minutes following the dynamic acquisition, planar images are taken in the anterior, posterior, right lateral, and left lateral positions at 500K counts per projection.

Radionuclide cerebrospinal fluid imaging (cisternograms)

Radionuclide cisternography is performed for the assessment of normal and abnormal drainage of cerebrospinal fluid, evaluation of hydrocephalus, and localization of leaking cerebrospinal fluid in the ears or nose. The procedure is performed by administration of In-111 DTPA via lumbar puncture by a licensed radiologist. Immediately following the lumbar puncture, a static image should be obtained to ensure proper administration of the isotope. Serial static images are then performed in the anterior, posterior, right lateral, and left lateral positions at 2, 6, 24, and 48 hours post-injection. Occasionally, images are obtained at 72 hours post-injection if deemed necessary by the interpreting radiologist. All images should be obtained for 100K counts or a maximum of 600 seconds per image.

Brain PET scan

A brain PET scan may be obtained to assess cerebral infarcts, differentiate depression from dementia, evaluate disorders of the basal ganglia such as Parkinson's disease and Huntington's disease, localize epileptic trigger points, and evaluate the location, extent, and recurrence of brain tumors. This technique may also be used to evaluate the effectiveness of therapeutic drugs used to treat mental illness.

Brain SPECT study

A brain SPECT study may be used to evaluate cerebrovascular disorders such as hemorrhages and TIA. This technique may also be used to evaluate psychiatric disorders like dementia. Brain SPECT is useful in evaluating head trauma and epilepsy, as well. The brain SPECT study is obtained following intravenous administration of Tc-99m HMPAO. The SPECT images are obtained by placing the patient on the imaging table in a supine position. The acquisition parameters are a complete 360-degree rotation for 64 frames at an imaging time that would allow approximately 200K counts per frame. A 128 x 128 matrix should be used for the acquisition.

Ga-67 imaging

Gallium studies are used to evaluate infectious and inflammatory processes such as fever of unknown origin, respiratory infections such as tuberculosis, acquired immune deficiency syndrome (AIDS), and tumors associated with lymphoma. The study is obtained following intravenous injection of 5 to 10 mCi of Ga-67 citrate. If evaluating for infection, an early set of images are obtained at 6 hours post-injection. If evaluating tumors, imaging is performed later—at 48 to 72 hours post-injection. During each set of images, a whole body image should be obtained. Static images of the head, chest, abdomen, and pelvis are also obtained during each imaging session. Occasionally, views of the extremities or SPECT images may be obtained if requested by the interpreting radiologist. All static images should be obtained for 1,000K counts. The energies of the photons of Ga-67 are 184 keV and 296 keV, so a medium-energy collimator should be used for all image acquisitions.

In-111-labeled leukocytes and Tc-99m-labeled leukocytes

Imaging studies used to evaluate infections may be obtained by labeling white blood cells with In-111 or Tc-99m HMPAO. The procedure of tagging the white cells is the same for either isotope. The identical amount of blood is withdrawn from the patient and the isotope is administered via intravenous injection. Activities of the isotopes are different, however, with In-111-labeled leukocytes yielding approximately 0.5 mCi, whereas Tc-99m-labeled leukocytes yield approximately 20 mCi. Because of their higher activity, the latter are preferred when imaging the extremities. In-111-labeled leukocytes are preferred when assessing abdominal or kidney infection; the infection may be masked if

Tc-99m is used due to genitourinary excretion of the isotope.

In-vivo method for tagging red blood cells

With the in-vivo method, tagging occurs entirely inside the body. This method requires 2 intravenous injections. Initially, the patient is injected with 10 mg of cold pyrophosphate. The pyrophosphate must circulate inside the body for approximately 20 minutes to adequately tag the red blood cells. After 20 minutes, the patient is injected intravenously with 20 to 30 mCi of Tc-99m pertechnetate. The isotope should circulate in the body for approximately 10 minutes before imaging may occur. No patient preparation is required for in-vivo tagging of red blood cells.

In-vitro method for tagging red blood cells

With the in-vitro method, tagging occurs entirely outside the body. UltraTag is the primary pharmaceutical used to tag red blood cells. The procedure for in-vitro tagging requires 2 intravenous injections. Initially, 5 mL of blood is withdrawn from the patient and 1 to 3 mL is then deposited into the UltraTag kit vial. The blood and UltraTag combination should be allowed to mix for approximately 5 minutes with occasional gentle shaking of the vial. Once the 5-minute mix is complete, syringe 1 of the UltraTag labeling kit is injected into the vial containing blood and UltraTag and gently shaken. Immediately after syringe 1 has been injected into the mixture, add syringe 2 to the mixture and gently swirl. Once syringe 2 has been injected, add 25 to 35 mCi of Tc-99m pertechnetate to the mixture and allow it to sit for 20 minutes with occasional gentle shaking. Once the 20-minute time period has elapsed, administer the entire mixture to the patient via intravenous injection. No patient preparation is required for in-vitro tagging of red blood cells.

MUGA scan

A MUGA scan is often obtained to assess the contractility of the left ventricle. This study is of great importance for patients who are undergoing chemotherapy treatments that may be cardiotoxic. A MUGA scan is obtained by tagging red blood cells with Tc-99m pertechnetate. This procedure may be performed using either in-vivo or in-vitro red blood cell tagging techniques. Once the red blood cells have been tagged with Tc-99m pertechnetate, imaging may be performed. A MUGA scan involves the acquisition of 3 gated images of the heart at anterior, 45-degree, and left lateral projections. It should be noted the 45-degree projection could be adjusted to a different angle to represent proper separation of the left and right ventricle. Prior to imaging, the patient must be connected to a heart monitor so gating and wall motion can be assessed. Each of the 3 views should be acquired for either 4,000K counts or 600 acquired heartbeats. Either of these parameters should provide adequate images to assess the contractility of the left ventricle.

Adenosine role in cardiac stress testing

Adenosine is a pharmaceutical that may be used to perform stress testing in patients who are unable to exercise on a treadmill or stationary bicycle. Adenosine acts a vasodilator in the body, which means it increases the diameter of the blood vessels in order to increase blood flow to all parts of the body. The vasodilatory properties of adenosine simulate exercise in the body, and myocardial perfusion can be accurately assessed after intravenous infusion of adenosine.

<u>Adenosine side effect</u>
Intravenous adenosine acts as a vasodilator and simulates exercise in the body. During an intravenous adenosine infusion, a patient may experience a warm, flushed feeling all over the body. In addition, a patient may experience shortness of breath, sweating, coughing, and a decrease in blood pressure during the infusion. The most significant side effect a patient may experience is high-degree A-V heart block. Adenosine decreases electrical conduction through the A-V node, which may induce first-, second-, or even third-degree heart block during an adenosine-induced stress test. Episodes of heart block are usually transient and resolve spontaneously during the infusion. If heart block does not resolve, immediately discontinue the infusion of adenosine.

Dobutamine role in cardiac stress testing

Dobutamine is a pharmaceutical that may be used to perform stress testing in patients who are unable to exercise on a treadmill or stationary bicycle. Dobutamine is commonly used to improve cardiac function in patients with heart failure and cardiogenic shock. Dobutamine enables the heart rate and blood pressure to increase to the point that a diagnostic stress test can be obtained and accurate myocardial perfusion imaging can be performed.

Thallium-201 myocardial viability imaging

Myocardial viability imaging with Tl-201 is often performed to assess the presence or extent of myocardial damage following a myocardial infarction. This procedure is also used to assess patency of the coronary arteries immediately after cardiac bypass surgery. The procedure is only performed with the patient in a resting state; viability imaging is not done during stress testing. The patient is injected with 2 to 4 mCi of Tl-201 intravenously; immediately following administration of Tl-201, a SPECT myocardial perfusion image is obtained. Additional SPECT myocardial perfusion images are obtained at 6 hours and 24 hours post-injection. The delayed images are used to determine if the area of the myocardial infarction will absorb Tl-201 over time, which will determine myocardial viability.

Myocardial stress testing

Prior to myocardial stress testing, the patient is instructed to have nothing by mouth for a minimum of 4 hours. This is to ensure the heart is the most metabolically active organ in the body and the maximum amount of isotope will be taken up by the heart and not the stomach. For treadmill and dobutamine-induced stress tests, patients are instructed to discontinue any beta-blocker medications. Beta-blockers make it difficult to achieve maximum heart rate. For adenosine and regadenoson-induced stress tests, patients are instructed to discontinue any medications that contain theophylline and refrain from any food or beverage that may contain caffeine. Theophylline and caffeine counteract adenosine and regadenoson, which may result in an inadequate amount of stress on the heart. Diabetic patients should have their medications and diets adjusted by their primary care physician prior to cardiac stress testing.

Heart

The heart is comprised of 3 layers, the epicardium, myocardium, and endocardium. The epicardium is the thin, outermost layer. The myocardium is the thick, muscular, middle layer that is responsible for the majority of the pumping action of the ventricles. The innermost layer of the heart is the endocardium. The endocardium is responsible for overall cardiac function.

Myocardium cells

There are 2 types of cells in the myocardium: contractile cells, which make up the bulk of the myocardium, and electrical cells, which are made of specific excitatory and conductive fibers. The contractile cells cause the pumping action of the heart and the electrical cells are responsible for rapid conduction of impulses throughout the heart. These 2 types of cells work in conjunction with each other to keep the heart beating in a regular, rhythmic manner.

Cardiac PET imaging

Attenuation correction is crucial in PET imaging. The effects of attenuation are much more evident with PET than with SPECT because the 511 keV positrons are constantly being attenuated during their path between the 2 detectors. During SPECT imaging, the attenuation path is variable. But with PET imaging, that path is constant. Therefore, the algorithms used for attenuation correction during PET imaging are much more accurate than those used with SPECT imaging.

PET vs. SPECT

Compared to SPECT, PET scanning of the heart provides greater spatial and temporal resolution. PET imaging also exhibits greater attenuation and scatter correction, which enables better quantitative measurements such as absolute blood flow. In addition, PET allows for imaging during actual physical stress, which could identify stress-induced changes in cardiac function.

Cardiac PET scan

PET myocardial perfusion imaging may be performed if a patient has previously had a suboptimal, clinically inadequate cardiac SPECT study. If the patient has a large body habitus that makes it difficult to obtain optimal SPECT images, PET with attenuation correction can reduce the likelihood of a false-positive study. Evaluation of patients suspected of having multivessel coronary disease is improved with PET scanning because myocardial perfusion can be precisely quantified in milliliters per minute per gram of tissue.

N-13 role

N-13 has been used for research purposes for over 20 years and was just recently approved for clinical use. The half-life of N-13 is 10 minutes, which makes the isotope difficult to use in a clinical setting because an on-site cyclotron is required. However, image quality with N-13 is superior because 90% of the tracer localizes in the myocardium, leaving very little background in the images. N-13 is taken up in the myocardium in a fairly homogenous manner. The lateral wall of the left ventricle may appear slightly less perfused an artifact that occurs even in healthy patients. Gated wall motion analysis should help differentiate this artifact from a true perfusion defect.

Rb-82 role

Rb-82 is the most popular radiotracer for cardiac PET imaging. The half-life of Rb-82 is 75 seconds, but an on-site cyclotron is not required like it is with N-13. Rb-82 can be obtained from a generator similar to that of Tc-99m. Rb-82 is a potassium analog, so it is taken up in the myocardium via active transport. The uptake of Rb-82 in the myocardium is similar to that of the Tl-201 used for SPECT imaging, but less than that of N-13.

FDG (F-18) role

FDG which is a glucose analog is the gold standard for assessing myocardial viability. FDG has a half-life of 110 minutes, so a cyclotron is not required on-site. FDG has the highest spatial resolution of all positron emitters due to low kinetic energy of the positron. FDG is taken up in the myocardium via active transport and it competes with other forms of glucose in the body for transport in the myocardium. In a fasting patient, the myocardium would likely use more fatty acids than glucose. By injecting another form of glucose, the natural insulin response is for the myocardium to primarily use glucose instead of fatty acids.

N-13 cardiac PET protocol

N-13 is usually used in conjunction with a rest/stress cardiac protocol. Intravenous administration of 10 to 15 mCi of N-13 is required before both rest and stress image acquisitions. N-13 should be administered slowly over 20 to 30 seconds. It is rapidly taken up in the myocardium, usually within 90 seconds. Due to the short half-life of N-13, imaging should be started within 2 to 3 minutes of administration. Total scan time should ideally be from 5 to 15 minutes; image acquisitions over 20 minutes are usually not diagnostic due to the 10-minute half-life of N-13. A waiting period of 60 minutes should be allowed between rest and stress to allow 6 half-lives of tracer decay for optimal stress imaging. Lung uptake is common in patients who smoke or have congestive heart failure. Occasionally, there may be intense liver uptake, which can make the inferior wall difficult to interpret. If this occurs, the

time between injection and scan may need to be increased.

Rb-82 cardiac PET protocol

Rb-82 is usually used in conjunction with a rest/stress cardiac protocol. Intravenous administration of 40 to 60 mCi of Rb-82 is required before both rest and stress image acquisitions. For PET/CT imaging, a scout image should be performed before each acquisition to ensure proper patient position. It is critical to allow clearance of the blood pool before beginning either acquisition. This is because a high number of blood pool counts can make the left ventricle appear smaller on the rest images and thus falsely dilated on the stress images. For patients with normal left ventricular function, imaging may be initiated within 70 to 90 seconds. For patients with diminished left ventricular function, imaging may be delayed to 110 to 130 minutes.

FDG (F-18) cardiac viability PET protocol

FDG is used to assess myocardial viability. In order for myocardial viability to be assessed, myocardial perfusion must be assessed first. Ideally, perfusion should be assessed using Rb-82 or N-13 so comparison can be made with imaging performed on same piece of equipment. However, comparison can be made with traditional SPECT imaging. In order to obtain FDG images, the patient must fast for a minimum of 6 hours and then undergo a blood sugar test. Blood sugar should be between 100 and 140 mg/dL for optimal FDG imaging. The patient is then given 10 to 15 mCi of FDG intravenously. A minimum of 45 minutes should elapse between administration of FDG and imaging to allow for adequate blood pool clearance. Scan time is usually 10 to 30 minutes and attenuation correction should be performed. In addition, gating should be performed because wall motion is useful when determining myocardial viability.

Contraindications for thyroid imaging

The most important contraindication for thyroid imaging is medication. Patients should be instructed to discontinue all medications that directly affect the thyroid prior to thyroid imaging. Medications such as levothyroxine, which increases thyroid function, should be discontinued for 4 to 6 weeks prior to testing. Propylthiouracil (PTU) and methimazole are thyroid suppressants that should be discontinued for 7 days prior to testing. Patients who have had other diagnostic procedures involving the use of an intravenous iodine-based dye should wait 4 to 6 weeks to have thyroid imaging. The iodine dye will alter thyroid scan results if not allowed to clear the system for 4 to 6 weeks. Patients undergoing thyroid evaluation should also be instructed to stay away from any foods that contain high amounts of iodine, particularly seafood.

Thyroid uptake

A thyroid uptake is used to evaluate the function of the thyroid gland. An uptake is commonly used in conjunction with thyroid imaging, but can be performed alone if simply assessing hyperthyroidism or hypothyroidism. A thyroid uptake is performed using 200 to 600 µCi of iodine-123 or iodine-131. Prior to administration of the tracer to the patient, the iodine capsule must be counted using either an uptake probe or pinhole collimator. The counts of the capsule and room background must be recorded prior to administration of the iodine capsules. The patient must also be questioned to check for contraindications before the iodine capsules are administered. Uptakes are usually completed at 6 hours and 24 hours after administration. Using an uptake probe or pinhole collimator, these uptakes are performed by obtaining counts of the thyroid for 1 to 2 minutes and then recording the number of counts. A standard, usually the thigh, should also be counted for 1 to 2 minutes and the number of counts should be recorded. The thigh is used because it is normally similar to the neck in size, shape, and geometry and provides an accurate body background. The formula for calculating thyroid uptake is:

$$Thyroid\ uptake\ \% = \frac{Thyroid\ counts - Patient\ background\ counts\ (thigh)}{Capsule\ counts - Room\ background\ counts} \times 100\%$$

Thyroid imaging indicators

Thyroid imaging is performed to help differentiate between benign and malignant thyroid nodules. Imaging can be performed to assess the function of an individual nodule compared with the other parts of the thyroid gland. For conditions such as toxic nodular goiter, imaging may be performed to assess the homogeneity of the thyroid gland. Thyroid images are also obtained to assess for residual thyroid tissue after thyroidectomy and to assess for metastases from thyroid cancer.

Iodine-131 whole body imaging

Whole body imaging with iodine-131 is used to evaluate metastases from thyroid cancer. An I-131 whole body scan can be obtained by itself or in conjunction with high-dose iodine ablation of thyroid cancer. An I-131 whole body scan is performed following oral administration of 1 to 3 mCi of I-131. The scan parameters are similar to those of a whole body bone scan, but the scan speed should be slowed to account for lower activity. Images are acquired at 48 hours and 72 hours after administration of I-131. The views acquired should include a whole body scan with static images of the neck, chest, abdomen, and pelvis. All static images should be acquired for no less than 600 seconds. When used in conjunction with high-dose thyroid ablation, the identical views should be obtained 7 days after the ablation was performed.

Parathyroid glands

The parathyroid glands control and regulate the level of calcium in the body by producing and releasing parathyroid hormone (PTH). Low calcium levels in the body will stimulate production of parathyroid hormone from the parathyroid glands and stimulate calcium release from the skeleton, gastrointestinal tract, and kidneys. The parathyroid glands are different than the thyroid in that PTH is not stored within the glands, but is produced and released when stimulated by low calcium levels.

Detection of parathyroid adenomas

Parathyroid images can be obtained with 2 different methods: a dual isotope method using both Thallium-201 and Technetium-99m pertechnetate or a serial static imaging method using Technetium-99m sestamibi. Either protocol is adequate for the detection of parathyroid adenomas.

Parathyroid scan

Parathyroid scans are routinely performed to identify single parathyroid adenomas, multiple parathyroid adenomas, or glandular hyperplasia in patients who have a new diagnosis of hypocalcemia and elevated parathyroid hormone levels. Parathyroid scans can also be useful in shortening surgical time by accurately localizing parathyroid adenomas before surgery. In addition, parathyroid imaging is useful in localizing parathyroid tissue in patients with recurrent hyperparathyroidism after surgical intervention.

Dual isotope procedure for parathyroid imaging

The dual isotope parathyroid protocol begins with an intravenous injection of 2 to 3 mCi of TI-201. Within 2 to 3 minutes of injection, imaging should begin. If using a high-resolution collimator, obtain a static image for 600 seconds on a 256x256x16 matrix. The detector should be positioned with the thyroid gland at the top and the heart at the bottom of the field of view. If using a pinhole collimator, 2 views may be needed to accurately evaluate for parathyroid adenomas; one should be obtained with the field of view centered on the upper mediation between the thyroid and the heart, and the other with the thyroid in the center of the field of view. Pinhole images should be acquired for 900 seconds on a 256x256x16 matrix. Once the thallium images have been obtained, 5 to 10 mCi of Tc-99m pertechnetate should be administered intravenously. After a 5-minute waiting period to allow for proper circulation of Tc-99m, obtain identical views with the identical parameters used with Tl-201. Process the images by serial subtraction of the Tc-99m images from the TI-201 images until the entire thyroid gland has been removed.

Parathyroid imaging using Tc-99m-sestamibi

Parathyroid images can be obtained by administering a single injection of Tc-99m sestamibi. The procedure begins with an intravenous injection of 20 to 30 mCi of

- 29 -

Tc-99m sestamibi. Allow approximately 10 minutes for proper circulation of the isotope; then use a high-resolution collimator to image the parathyroid glands. A static image should be obtained for 600 seconds on a 256x256x16 matrix. The image should be positioned with the thyroid at the top and the heart at the bottom of the field of view. Once the first static image is acquired, a second image should be obtained in identical position using identical parameters with a marker placed on the sternal notch. After the marker image is obtained, wait 2 hours to allow the Tc-99m sestamibi to washout of the thyroid gland. Then obtain a second set of identical images with identical parameters and compare the two sets of images. On the delayed images, any residual activity around the poles of the thyroid gland will indicate the presence of a parathyroid adenoma.

I-131 MIBG procedure indicators

I-131 MIBG is used to localize pheochromocytoma in patients who present with classic symptoms of the tumor or abnormal blood work indicating the presence of such a tumor. I-131MIBG studies are also obtained to evaluate for metastases from a previously diagnosed pheochromocytoma. Other neuroendocrine tumors such as neuroblastoma, medullary thyroid carcinoma, and Merkel cell tumors can also be diagnosed or evaluated with this procedure.

I-131 MIBG study

An I-131 MIBG study is initiated with an intravenous injection of 3 to 10 mCi of I-131 MIBG. The injection should be administered over approximately 15 seconds. Static images should be obtained at 4, 24, and 48 hours after the injection. Images may be obtained at 72 hours post-injection if required by the interpreting

physician. Static images should be acquired of the skull, chest, abdomen, and pelvis in both the anterior and posterior positions. Imaging of the femurs should also be performed if evaluating for metastases from an existing pheochromocytoma. All static images should be obtained for a minimum of 100K counts or a minimum of 20 minutes. SPECT images may also be obtained if required by the interpreting physician.

Gastric emptying study

A gastric emptying study is a noninvasive way to quantify gastric emptying. These studies are obtained to evaluate for delayed gastric emptying and quantify the rate of gastric emptying for individuals suspected of having gastric motility problems. Gastric emptying studies are also useful for determining the effectiveness of therapy for patients with known gastric motility problems.

Meals administered
The meal administered to obtain a gastric emptying study may vary by facility, depending on the preference of the interpreting physicians. The ideal meal for this procedure is a chicken liver labeled with Tc-99m sulfur colloid in vivo, although this method is cumbersome and virtually impossible to perform in a clinical setting. Therefore, the most common meal for evaluating gastric emptying is a Tc-99m sulfur colloid-labeled scrambled egg taken by mouth. Occasionally, patients presenting for gastric emptying studies have an allergy to eggs. In this case, Tc-99m sulfur colloid may be incorporated into a bowl of oatmeal.

Procedure
In order for a gastric emptying study to be accurate, the patient must be NPO for at least 8 hours prior to the procedure. The procedure begins with ingestion of the

radioactive meal containing approximately 1 mCi of Tc-99m sulfur colloid. The patient should be instructed to eat the meal in approximately 5 minutes so imaging can begin as soon as possible. This may consist of serial static imaging or dynamic imaging. If using serial static imaging, images should be obtained every 15 minutes for 2 hours. This should include 60 seconds of images with the patient in the erect position. If using a dynamic protocol, imaging should be set for 120 images at 60 seconds each for a total of 120 minutes. During dynamic imaging, the patient should be in the supine position with the detector placed over the abdomen.

Gastroesophageal reflux study indicators

A gastroesophageal reflux study may be obtained when patients present with symptoms of gastrointestinal reflux such as chest pain or vomiting. This study may be indicated in children if aspiration is expected. It is also effective for evaluating the response of gastroesophageal reflux to a medical or a surgical intervention.

Procedure for performing a gastroesophageal reflux study in adults
To ensure an accurate gastroesophageal reflux study, adult patients should be NPO for at least 8 hours prior to the procedure. The study begins with the patient drinking a mixture of 150 mL of orange juice, 150 mL of 0.1N hydrochloric acid, and approximately 300 µCi of Tc-99m sulfur colloid. Then, an abdominal binder is immediately placed on the patient and a static image is obtained for 30 seconds using a 64x64 matrix with the patient in the erect position. After the immediate static image, the abdominal binder is inflated to a pressure of 20 mm/Hg and additional static images are obtained. This process is repeated at each 20 mm/Hg increment until a maximum abdominal binder pressure of 100 mm/Hg is reached. The abdominal binder is then rapidly deflated to release the pressure on the abdominal wall and the procedure is repeated with the patient in the supine position.

Procedure for performing a gastroesophageal reflux study in children
When having a gastroesophageal reflux study, a child should be NPO and the procedure should ideally be performed in conjunction with the child's normal feeding time. With the child semi-recumbent and his or her back to the camera with the mouth and stomach both in the field of view, the child ingests a mixture of approximately 150 µCi of Tc-99m sulfur colloid and 30 mL of milk or baby formula. While the child is drinking, a dynamic acquisition is obtained at 2 seconds per frame for a total of 120 seconds. Once the feeding is complete, unlabeled milk or baby formula is administered to rinse the mouth and esophagus. The child is then placed in the supine position and an additional dynamic study is performed at 60 seconds per frame for a total of 60 minutes. Static images are then acquired in the anterior and posterior positions for 300 seconds to check the lungs for aspiration. Additional imaging may be performed at 2 hours and 24 hours to further evaluate the lungs for aspiration.

Esophageal transit imaging indicators

Esophageal transit imaging is used primarily for the diagnosis of dysphagia or any other abnormality with esophageal motility. Esophageal transit imaging can accurately quantify these abnormalities, even if they are secondary to other conditions such as achalasia, scleroderma, esophageal spasm, or reflux esophagitis.

Esophageal transit study procedures

To ensure accuracy in an esophageal transit study, the patient should be NPO for a minimum of 8 hours. A liquid preparation of 30 mL of water is combined with approximately 300 µCi of Tc-99m sulfur colloid. An esophageal transit study is a two-phase dynamic study. The initial swallow phase is acquired for 1 second per frame for 60 seconds. The second phase, or washout phase, is acquired for 15 seconds per frame for 10 minutes for a total study time of 11 minutes. The study begins when the patient is instructed to turn his or her head to one side to allow for ingestion of the water and sulfur colloid mixture. The patient sips the mixture through a straw and holds it in his or her mouth without swallowing. At this time, the dynamic acquisition is begun. Once the acquisition is started, the patient is instructed to swallow the mixture and then to dry swallow every 15 seconds for the remainder of the 11-minute study.

Meckel's diverticulum

Meckel's diverticulum is a congenital birth defect that manifests as a pouch on the wall of the lower part of the small bowel. The pouch may contain stomach tissue or pancreatic tissue. Symptoms of Meckel's diverticulum include mild to severe abdominal discomfort and blood in the stool. The symptoms usually occur during childhood but may not occur until adulthood. If bleeding develops, surgical intervention to remove the diverticulum is recommended.

Meckel's diverticulum study

A Meckel's diverticulum study is performed to localize the site of a Meckel's diverticulum that is causing gastrointestinal bleeding. Meckel's diverticulum is difficult to diagnose with other imaging modalities such as barium enemas. Tc-99m pertechnetate will localize a Meckel's diverticulum that contains stomach tissue. Most bleeding Meckel's diverticula contain such tissue.

Procedures
To ensure an accurate Meckel's diverticulum study, the patient should be NPO for a minimum of 4 hours. Infants should miss one feeding before the procedure is performed. The dose of Tc-99m pertechnetate is 15 mCi for adults and 200 µCi per kilogram with a minimum dose of 2 mCi for children. The patient should be instructed to empty the bladder completely immediately prior to intravenous administration of Tc-99m pertechnetate. Once the isotope is administered, 1,000K static images of the abdomen are obtained immediately and then every 5 minutes for 60 minutes. The images are acquired using a 256x256x16 matrix. After 60 minutes, the patient is instructed to completely empty the bladder once again; 60-minute post-void anterior and lateral images are then obtained using the same parameters.

GI bleeding procedure

A GI bleeding procedure is performed to localize the site of an active GI bleed so it can be surgically corrected. The primary indication for this procedure is the presence of blood in the stool. Other indications may include dark, tarry stools and low hemoglobin/hematocrit levels.

Procedures
GI bleeding procedures involve the labeling of red blood cells with Tc-99m pertechnetate using either the in vivo or in vitro method. GI bleeding studies are performed using a dynamic acquisition of 60-second frames for 60 minutes. The patient should be in a supine position with the detector over the abdomen. The trace is then injected intravenously and

the dynamic acquisition is begun. After 60 minutes, the patient may be instructed to void so an additional 1,000K static images can be obtained, if requested by the interpreting physician.

Hepatobiliary imaging

Hepatobiliary imaging is performed to diagnose acute cholecystitis, evaluate gallbladder function in patients with chronic cholecystitis, and assess for biliary leakage in post-surgical patients. The symptoms of these disorders are most commonly right upper-quadrant abdominal pain, nausea, and vomiting. Some patients describe symptoms of back pain, flank pain, or side pain.

Acute cholecystitis

Acute cholecystitis is defined as a sudden inflammation of the gallbladder that causes severe abdominal pain. Acute cholecystitis is usually caused by gallstones, although severe illnesses and gallbladder tumors may also lead to acute cholecystitis. Acute cholecystitis causes bile to become trapped in the gallbladder, which creates irritation and pressure inside the gallbladder. If acute cholecystitis is not diagnosed in a timely manner, serious infection or perforation of the gallbladder may result.

Chronic cholecystitis

Chronic cholecystitis is defined as a long-term swelling and inflammation of the gallbladder. Chronic cholecystitis is usually the product of repeated attacks of acute cholecystitis. Chronic cholecystitis ultimately leads to thickened gallbladder walls, shrinking the gallbladder itself and inhibiting the overall function of the gallbladder.

Cholecystokinin

Cholecystokinin is a hormone produced by the small intestine in response to the presence of fats that cause contraction of the gallbladder, the release of bile, and secretion of pancreatic digestive enzymes. Cholecystokinin belongs to a group of medicines known as diagnostic aids which help to diagnose certain medical issues. Cholecystokinin is administered during procedures evaluating gallbladder and pancreatic function. Doses of Cholecystokinin vary according to body weight.

Contraindications for hepatobiliary imaging

Eating is one contraindication to hepatobiliary imaging. For a hepatobiliary study to be accurate, the patient should be NPO for no less than 6 hours. Eating prior to hepatobiliary imaging will contract the gallbladder, leading to a false-positive study. Opiate pain medication use is also a contraindication to hepatobiliary imaging. Opiate medications such as morphine and hydromorphone cause the Sphincter of Oddi and common bile duct to contract, resulting in delayed emptying of bile through the common bile duct. In addition, morphine and Dilaudid may cause bile to fill the gallbladder by increasing pressure of the Sphincter of Oddi, leading to a false-negative result for acute cholecystitis.

Hepatobiliary study procedures

To ensure an accurate hepatobiliary study, the patient should be NPO and should not have received any opiate pain medication for at least 6 hours prior to the procedure. Hepatobiliary imaging is performed after intravenous administration of 4 to 6 mCi of Tc-99m Choletec, mebrofenin, or disofenin. Once

Tc-99m has been administered, serial static images are obtained. The detector should be placed over the abdomen with the liver in the center of the field of view. Static images are obtained every 5 minutes for 60 minutes. Images are acquired for approximately 500K counts each. Over the 60 minutes of imaging, it should be possible to visualize activity in the liver, gallbladder, and small intestines. The inability to visualize activity in any one of these structures indicates a biliary obstruction and a positive hepatobiliary scan. Delayed images may be obtained at the request of the interpreting physician to ensure proper diagnosis.

Liver/spleen imaging

Liver/spleen imaging is indicated for diagnosis of hepatomegaly, splenomegaly and other abdominal masses. The procedure is also useful for pre-operative evaluation of liver metastases in patients with known malignancies and for evaluating patients with liver diseases such as cirrhosis and hepatitis. In addition, liver/spleen imaging can be used to evaluate trauma patients for liver rupture or hematoma.

Procedures
Liver/spleen imaging is performed following intravenous administration of 6 to 10 mCi of Tc-99m sulfur colloid. There are no patient preparations for the exam. However, a past history of studies involving barium ingestion may be associated with false-positive results due to the presence of barium in the colon. After isotope administration, a 10-minute waiting period should be allowed to ensure proper uptake into the liver and spleen. Then a series of 600K to 1,000K static liver and spleen images are obtained on a 256x256x16 matrix. The views that are acquired include anterior, anterior with a liver marker, posterior, right lateral, left lateral, right anterior

oblique, and left anterior oblique. Posterior oblique images and SPECT scanning may also be performed at the request of the interpreting physician.

Hepatic hemangioma

Hepatic hemangioma is an abnormal, non-cancerous tumor in the liver that consists of dilated blood vessels. Hepatic hemangioma may cause abnormal bleeding and can even affect the function of the liver. Hepatic hemangiomas are most common in people 30 to 50 years of age. Women are more susceptible to hepatic hemangioma than men.

Hepatic hemangioma study

A hepatic hemangioma study begins with intravenous injection of Tc-99m-labeled red blood cells. The red blood cell tagging method can either be in vitro using UltraTag or in vivo using PYP. The dose of Tc-99m is 25 to 35 mCi. A hepatic hemangioma study consists of a dynamic phase, static imaging, and SPECT imaging if required. Review of an abdominal CT scan is necessary prior to injection of Tc-99m-labeled RBC's to ensure proper location of suspected hemangioma so the dynamic study is performed in the proper orientation. Once the location of suspected hemangioma is known, proceed with injection of labeled red blood cells and begin the dynamic phase. Acquire the dynamic phase for 60 frames at 4 seconds per frame using a 64x64x16 matrix. Once the dynamic phase is complete, immediately begin static imaging. Acquire static images in the anterior, posterior, and right lateral positions. Each static image should be acquired for at least 1,000k counts using a 256x256x16 matrix. After the immediate static images are obtained, there is a 2-hour waiting period before a second set of images is obtained. Acquire the second set in the identical anterior, posterior, and

- 34 -

right lateral positions. An abdominal SPECT may be necessary if the interpreting radiologist needs additional information to make an accurate diagnosis.

Furosemide role in renal studies

Furosemide is a medication prescribed to reduce swelling, urine retention, and high blood pressure. It stimulates the kidneys to increase urine output to rid the body of excess water and salts. Furosemide is commonly administered during renal scans to evaluate flow and function of the kidneys in response to furosemide stimulation. A normal renogram will reveal increased flow and function in both kidneys in response to furosemide administration.

Procedure

A furosemide renal scan can be obtained following the intravenous administration of 10 to 15 mCi of either Tc-99m MAG3 or Tc-99m DTPA. An intravenous catheter should be inserted to ensure complete administration of the isotope and no chance for extravasation of the injection. Prior to injection, the patient should be placed on the imaging table in the supine position with the camera in the posterior position. To ensure proper positioning of the patient, the landmarks of the xiphoid process and symphysis pubis should be marked to ensure the kidneys are in field of view. The renal scan is performed using a 2-phase dynamic protocol. Following the administration of Tc-99m MAG3 or DTPA, an initial flow dynamic phase should be acquired for 60 frames at 1 second per frame using a 64x64x16 matrix. Immediately following the initial flow dynamic, a functional dynamic phase should be acquired for 180 frames at 15 seconds per frame using a 64x64x16 matrix for a total of 46 minutes of imaging time. Approximately 10 minutes after the study has begun, 40 mg of furosemide

should be administered intravenously by a nurse. It should be noted that furosemide will increase kidney function and urine output; some patients may not be able to tolerate the entire 46-minute procedure because the urge to urinate may be too great.

Captopril role in renal studies

Captopril belongs to a group of medicines known as ACE inhibitors. It is often used to treat high blood pressure and congestive heart failure. Captopril has a specific affect on the kidneys and is often administered prior to renal studies to evaluate a renal artery blockage. A captopril renal study will reveal a slight increase in renal function if the kidneys are not blocked and a decrease in renal function if renal artery blockage is present.

Captopril renal scan

A captopril renal scan can be obtained following the intravenous administration of 10 to 15 mCi of either Tc-99m MAG3 or Tc-99m DTPA. An intravenous catheter should be inserted to ensure complete administration of the isotope and no chance for extravasation of the injection. In order to obtain the desired renal effect, 25 to 50 mg of captopril should be administered orally 1 hour prior to the study. The patient's blood pressure should be monitored every 15 minutes after captopril administration since captopril may cause hypotension. Prior to injection, the patient should be placed on the imaging table in the supine position with the camera in the posterior position. To ensure proper positioning of the patient, the landmarks of the xiphoid process and symphysis pubis should be marked to ensure kidneys are in field of view. The renal scan is performed using a 2-phase dynamic protocol. Following the administration of Tc-99m MAG3 or DTPA, an initial flow dynamic phase should be acquired for 60 frames at 1 second per frame using a 64x64x16 matrix. Immediately following the initial flow dynamic, a functional dynamic phase should be acquired for 180 frames at 15 seconds per frame using a 64x64x16 matrix for a total of 46 minutes of imaging time.

Renal scan

Renal scans are performed to evaluate overall kidney function either in native or transplanted kidneys. Renal scans are particularly useful in evaluating glomerular filtration rate and renal plasma flow, diagnosing renal artery and ureteral obstruction, and assessing patients with suspected renovascular hypertension.

Renogram procedures

A renogram can be obtained following the intravenous administration of 10 to 15 mCi of either Tc-99m MAG3 or Tc-99m DTPA. An intravenous catheter should be inserted to ensure complete administration of the isotope and no chance for extravasation of the injection. Prior to injection, the patient should be placed on the imaging table in the supine position with the camera in the posterior position. To ensure proper positioning of the patient, the landmarks of the xiphoid process and symphysis pubis should be marked to ensure the kidneys are in field of view. The renal scan is performed using a 2-phase dynamic protocol. Following the administration of Tc-99m MAG3 or DTPA, an initial flow dynamic phase should be acquired for 60 frames at 1 second per frame using a 64x64x16 matrix.

Immediately following the initial flow dynamic, a functional dynamic phase should be acquired for 120 frames at 15

seconds per frame using a 64x64x16 matrix for a total of 31 minutes of imaging time.

Lung perfusion imaging

Lung perfusion imaging is primarily performed to evaluate patients for pulmonary embolism. Lung perfusion imaging is also performed in patients with known pulmonary emboli to evaluate the progress of the treatment regimen used to dissolve the emboli. Alterations in lung perfusion caused by lung malignancies, emphysema, chronic bronchitis and asthma can also be evaluated using lung perfusion imaging.

Lung ventilation images

Lung ventilation imaging can be obtained with either Xe-133 gas or Tc-99m DTPA aerosol. To obtain Xe-133 images, a closed ventilation system and negative room pressure are required in case of accidental release of Xe-133 into the room. To obtain lung ventilation images using Tc-99m DTPA aerosol, a nebulizer is required to convert the Tc-99m DTPA from liquid form to aerosolized droplet form. Tc-99m DTPA aerosol is the most common method of obtaining lung ventilation images because negative room pressure is not required, thus reducing costs for the facility.

Xe-133
The first step in lung ventilation imaging with Xe-133 is to turn on the exhaust system in the negative-pressure room in case of accidental release of Xe-133. Position the patient in front of the detector in the posterior position; then securely attach the facemask to the patient so it covers both the nose and mouth. Xe-133 imaging is performed using a dynamic protocol. The computer should be programmed for 32 frames at 15 seconds per frame for a total of 8

minutes of imaging. Instruct the patient to take a deep breath. As he or she does so, simultaneously administer 10 to 15 mCi of Xe-133 and begin the dynamic acquisition. Instruct the patient to hold his or her breath for the first 15 seconds so an initial deep-breathing image can be obtained. The patient should then be instructed to breathe normally for the remainder of the procedure. At this time, the majority of the Xe-133 should be eliminated from the lungs. Finally, turn off the xenon delivery system and remove the patient's facemask.

Tc-99m DTPA

A nebulizer is required to convert Tc-99m DTPA from liquid to aerosol form. Initially, 30 to 40 mCi of Tc-99m DTPA should be inserted into the nebulizer. Attach oxygen tubing to the nebulizer, but do not turn the oxygen on until the patient is ready to breathe (to avoid contamination). Tc-99m aerosol can be administered through a facemask or mouthpiece and nose clip. Instruct the patient to insert the mouthpiece or apply the facemask tightly so it covers the nose and mouth. Turn the oxygen on to 12 to 15 liters to ensure proper aerosol droplet size. Instruct the patient to breathe normally for 4 to 5 minutes without taking out the mouthpiece or removing the facemask. Then remove the mouthpiece or facemask and begin static imaging with the patient on the imaging table in the supine position. Ventilation images are routinely acquired for 150K to 250K counts using a 128x128x16 matrix. Static images are routinely acquired in the anterior, right lateral, right posterior oblique, posterior, left posterior oblique and left lateral positions. Right anterior oblique and left anterior oblique images may also be obtained if requested by the interpreting physician.

Quantitative lung perfusion imaging

Quantitative lung imaging is often performed prior to surgical procedures such as pneumonectomy or lung reduction. Quantitative lung imaging is obtained via intravenous injection of 4 to 6 mCi of Tc-99m MAA. To ensure even distribution of Tc-99m MAA particles in the lungs, the patient should be placed on the imaging table in the supine position prior to intravenous injection. After the injection, a series of static images are obtained. Quantitative imaging routinely consists of static images acquired in the anterior, posterior, right lateral, left lateral, right posterior oblique and left posterior oblique positions. Anterior oblique images can also be obtained if requested by the interpreting physician. All images should be acquired using 256x256x16 matrix. The anterior and posterior images should be acquired for 1,000K counts and all other images for 500K counts. Once static images are acquired, the images are ready to be processed. Regions of interest should be drawn around each lung on both the anterior and posterior projections. The processing software should calculate the number of counts in each lobe of the lung. If using older processing software, regions of interest may need to be drawn around each lobe of the lung to achieve desired results.

Lung ventilation/perfusion imaging

Lung ventilation/perfusion imaging is very commonly used to diagnose pulmonary embolism. Initially, 30 - 40 mCi of Tc-99m DTPA should be inserted into the nebulizer. Attach oxygen tubing to the nebulizer, but do not turn the oxygen on until the patient is ready to breathe (to avoid contamination). Tc-99m aerosol can be administered through a facemask or mouthpiece and nose clip. Instruct the patient to insert the mouthpiece or apply the facemask tightly so it covers the nose and mouth. Turn the oxygen on to 12 to 15 liters to ensure proper aerosol droplet size. Instruct patient to breathe normally for 4 to 5 minutes without taking out the mouthpiece or removing the facemask. Then remove the mouthpiece or facemask and begin static imaging with the patient on the imaging table in the supine position. Ventilation images are routinely acquired for 150K to 250K counts using a 128x128x16 matrix. Static images are routinely acquired in the anterior, right lateral, right posterior oblique, posterior, left posterior oblique and left lateral positions. Right anterior oblique and left anterior oblique images may also be obtained if requested by the interpreting physician. Once ventilation images have been obtained, an intravenous injection of 4 to 6 mCi of Tc-99m MAA is administered. Perfusion images are then obtained in the identical positions as the ventilation images. Perfusion images are acquired for 500K counts using a 256x256x16 matrix.

Breast imaging

Breast imaging is routinely performed after a non-diagnostic mammogram to identify sites of malignancy within the breast or sites of metastasis from known primary breast carcinoma. Breast imaging can be obtained with Tl-201 or Tc-99m sestamibi. Tc-99m sestamibi is the isotope of choice primarily because it is taken up in the identical sites as Tl-201, but with much higher count rates and resolution.

Procedure
Breast images are obtained via intravenous injection of 3 mCi of Tl-201 or 25 mCi of Tc-99m sestamibi. It should be noted that the injection should occur in the arm opposite the suspected malignancy. For example, if the suspected

malignancy is in the left breast, inject the isotope into the right arm. Allow approximately 5 minutes for proper circulation of the isotope. Then initiate static imaging with the patient on the imaging table in the supine position and the arms placed above the head. Static images should be acquired for 300 to 600 seconds using a 256x256x16 matrix. The armpit and breast should be included in the field of view. Cobalt disk markers should be placed in the armpit area and in the area of the suspected malignancy. The breasts should be positioned to avoid overlapping of the liver or heart. Images are acquired in the anterior, right anterior oblique and left anterior oblique positions. SPECT imaging may also be performed if required by the interpreting physician.

LeVeen shunt

A LeVeen shunt is a device used to remove excess fluid from the peritoneal cavity. This fluid, also known as ascites, is commonly found in patients with cirrhosis of the liver. The LeVeen shunt is inserted into the peritoneal cavity and drains into the superior vena cava through a venous tube placed in the jugular vein. The venous tube has a one-way valve that opens when the pressure of the fluid in the peritoneal cavity is greater than the pressure in the superior vena cava.

LeVeen shunt study procedure

The LeVeen shunt study is performed to evaluate the proper functioning of a LeVeen shunt. The study is performed via intraperitoneal injection 2 to 5 mCi Tc-99m MAA. It should be noted that a nuclear medicine technologist is not permitted to perform the intraperitoneal injection; this must be performed by a licensed radiologist. Prior to intraperitoneal injection, the patient must

- 38 -

be placed on the imaging table in the supine position. The patient's abdomen must then be cleansed in a sterile manner using Betadine. The radiologist then administers 2 to 5 mCi of Tc-99 MAA directly in to the peritoneum. Immediately following injection, static images of the chest and abdomen are acquired for 1,000K counts using a 256x256x16 matrix. Serial static images should be acquired every 15 minutes for 60 minutes. Delayed images are occasionally required at 2 hours or 4 hours post-injection. The study is complete and considered normal when the lungs become visible. If the lungs do not visualize, the study is considered positive and the shunt is considered dysfunctional.

Radionuclide cisternography

Radionuclide cisternography is performed to evaluate the flow of cerebrospinal fluid though the spinal column. Cisternography is also used to evaluate hydrocephalus and the associated shunting, to assess the patency of a shunt inserted to decrease hydrocephalus-related pressure, and to diagnose and localize cerebrospinal fluid leaks such as rhinorrhea or otorrhea.

Procedure
Cisternography is obtained via intrathecal injection (lumbar puncture) of 1 mCi of In-111 DTPA. It should be noted that nuclear medicine technologists are not permitted to administer In-111 DTPA via lumbar puncture; this should be performed by a licensed radiologist. Prior to the lumbar puncture, the patient is placed on the imaging table in the fetal position to allow the disc spaces to open and facilitate lumbar puncture and isotope administration. The physician then cleanses the patient's back and administers the isotope. Immediately following the lumbar puncture, place the

patient on the imaging table in the supine position and acquire a 100K-count or 600-second static image to ensure proper location of the isotope. The images should be acquired using a 128x128x16 matrix. Static images should then be obtained at 2, 6, 24 and 48 hours after isotope administration in the anterior, right lateral and left lateral positions using the identical parameters. Imaging may be taken out to 72 hours post-injection if required by the interpreting physician.

Dose calibrator linearity testing

Linearity testing of the dose calibrator is performed to ensure the dose calibrator accurately calibrates every dose regardless of the activity of the dose. The dose calibrator should calibrate radioactivity at levels of 200 mCi and higher as accurately as it measures radioactivity at levels as low as 10 µCi. Dose calibrator linearity evaluations should be performed immediately upon receipt of the equipment and quarterly thereafter. Linearity evaluations can be performed with the decay method or the Calicheck method. Either method will accurately determine linearity for the piece of equipment.

Decay method
The decay method begins with a dose of Tc-99m pertechnetate equal to or greater than the highest activity that will be administered to the patient. For laboratories performing therapy procedures, this could be as high as 200 mCi. Record a background reading for the dose calibrator. Then record the reading of the Tc-99m dose, subtract the background reading, and document the value obtained. Repeat this several times throughout the day at 1 to 2 hour increments and document the values. Continue to obtain readings until the original dose of Tc-99m pertechnetate has decayed to approximately 10 µCi. Once all

values have been obtained and recorded, calculate the expected readings for all documented times using the decay formula. On a piece of semi-log graph paper, plot the 2 lines of the actual readings against the calculated readings. All actual readings should be within 10% of calculated readings. If 1 value falls out of the 10% range, the dose calibrator should be repaired or replaced.

Calicheck method

The Calicheck method is the preferred method dose calibrator testing because it takes much less time and there is much less handling of a radioactive source, which in keeping with the ALARA principles. The Calicheck method requires a Calicheck kit, which consists of six lead-covered tubes used to simulate radioactive decay. The linearity evaluation begins with a dose of Tc-99m pertechnetate equal to or greater than the highest activity that will be administered to the patient. For laboratories performing therapy procedures, this could be as high as 200 mCi. Record a background reading for the dose calibrator. Then record the reading of the Tc-99m dose, subtract the background reading, and document the value obtained. Repeat the readings with each of the 6 lead-covered tubes and document the values. Once all values have been obtained and recorded, calculate the expected readings for all documented times using the decay formula. On a piece of semi-log graph paper, plot the 2 lines of the actual readings against the calculated readings. All actual readings should be within 10% of calculated readings. If 1 value falls out of the 10% range, the dose calibrator should be repaired or replaced.

Dose calibrator geometry evaluations

Geometry evaluations of the dose calibrator are critical to ensure the calibrator is accurately calibrating radioactivity, regardless of the volume of the sample. Ideally, a 10 mCi dose of radioactivity should be calibrated at 10 mCi whether it is in 1 mL or 30 mL of volume. If there is a discrepancy of the readings at various volumes, a correction factor may be applied to ensure accurate readings of the doses at various volumes. For example, if a 10 mCi dose of radioactivity gives a reading of 9 mCi when diluted into 30 mL of volume, a correction factor should be applied anytime a dose is measured in 30 mL. Geometric evaluations should be performed immediately upon receipt of the piece of equipment and immediately upon repair of the piece of equipment. This evaluation is NOT required quarterly like linearity testing.

Procedure
Begin a dose calibrator geometry evaluation by obtaining a 30-mL vial, then adding a small amount of volume and a small amount of radioactivity. The radioactive dose can vary, but it should be less than 10 mCi in approximately 1 mL of volume to begin geometric evaluation. Record the initial reading of the sample. Then continuously add volume to the sample in increments such as 5, 10, 15, 20, 25, and 30 mL and record the readings obtained for each volume. Ideally, the readings should be the same at all volumes. A correction factor needs to be applied if the readings vary. A correction factor is calculated with the following formula.

If the 15-mL volume reads 10.2 mCi when it should be reading no more than 10 mCi, the following calculation should be applied:

15-mL volume CF = 10 ÷ 10.2 = 0.98

For all 15-mL volumes, a correction factor of 0.98 should be applied.

Dose calibrator accuracy testing

Dose calibrator accuracy evaluations help to ensure that dose calibrators accurately read the activity of several different isotopes with several different energies. This evaluation should involve at least 2 different isotopes, such as Cs-137, Co-57 or Ba-133. These isotopes should be in the form of reference standards with known activities. Accuracy testing is required upon receipt of the piece of equipment and annually thereafter.

<u>Procedure</u>
Dose calibrator accuracy testing is performed using at least 2 different isotopes, such as Cs-137, Co-57 or Ba-133. These isotopes should be in the form of reference standards with known activities. The activity and date of calibration should be recorded on the reference vials. Calculate the current activity of the reference vials using the decay formula. A background reading should be recorded prior to accuracy testing. Assay the first reference vial, subtract the background reading, and document the final result. Repeat the reading 2 more times for a total of 3 readings and document the findings. Next, average the 3 readings. If the average of the actual readings differs from the calculated current activity by more than 10%, the dose calibrator should be repaired or replaced. Repeat this entire procedure for the second reference vial.

Dose calibrator constancy testing

Dose calibrator constancy testing should be performed on a daily basis to measure of the consistency of the piece of equipment. A long-lived isotope, such as Cs-137, should be used to perform the test so the readings can be reproducible from day to day over a long period of time.

<u>Procedure</u>
Constancy testing should be performed on a daily basis before any patient doses are assayed. A long-lived radioactivity source, such as Cs-137, should be used to perform constancy testing for the readings to be reproducible from one day to the next. Begin constancy testing by documenting the room background reading for the day. The high-voltage reading for the dose calibrator should also be recorded. Place the Cs-137 source in the dose calibrator and record the reading while the calibrator is set for Cs-137. Readings should also be recorded on all dose calibrator isotope settings that are commonly used in nuclear medicine. Tc-99m, Co-57, Ga-67, I-123, I-131, In-111 and Tl-201 should all be among the dose calibrator settings recorded in daily constancy evaluations.

Concert CPM to DPM

Converting counts per minute to disintegrations per minute is critical in the fields of nuclear medicine and health physics. The Department of Environmental Protection and other governing agencies require readings to be recorded in DPM rather than CPM. In order to convert CPM to DPM, the efficiency of the equipment being used must be known. Once the equipment efficiency is known, the following formula is used for the conversion.

$$Disintegrations\ per\ minute\ (DPM) = \frac{Counts\ per\ minute\ (CPM)}{Efficiency}$$

Example: A wipe test reading is 1,500 counts per minute and the efficiency of the well counter is 88%. What is the reading in DPM?

$$\frac{1500}{0.88} = 1705$$

Daily quality control procedures

The well counter should be calibrated and a background reading should be recorded. The uptake probe should be calibrated and a background reading should be recorded. All gamma cameras should be flooded to check for uniformity imperfections and flood images should be saved. A constancy evaluation should be performed on the dose calibrator. A daily department survey should be performed in all areas in which radioactive materials are used. A wipe test should be performed on all incoming radioactive shipments.

Instrumentation and Quality Control

Food field uniformity

Flood field uniformity refers to an imaging system's ability to produce a uniform diagnostic image. The uniformity of all nuclear medicine cameras should be evaluated prior to the start of every work day. A non-uniform area may show up as a "*hot*" or "*cold*" spot. These abnormalities could drastically affect nuclear medicine images and, in turn, the diagnosis based on those images. A "*hot*" spot could be read as a bone tumor, whereas a "*cold*" spot could be interpreted as a liver tumor. It is absolutely critical in nuclear medicine settings to ensure satisfactory uniformity of all nuclear medicine cameras before a patient image is obtained.

Evaluating extrinsic flood field uniformity

Flood field uniformity is most commonly evaluated in an extrinsic manner—i.e., with the collimator attached to the detector. A Co-57 sheet source is required to assess extrinsic uniformity. The use of a Co-57 sealed sheet source is beneficial because it greatly reduces the risk of radioactive contamination. Place the Co-57 sheet source directly onto a low-energy collimator. Acquire an image for approximately 15,000K counts using a 64x64x16 matrix. Once the image is obtained, it should be analyzed to ensure proper uniformity throughout the field of view.

Procedure

Intrinsic uniformity involves the evaluation of flood field uniformity with the collimator removed from the detector. This may be the desired method of evaluating flood filed uniformity if the cost of a sealed radioactive source is not in the budget. Intrinsic uniformity is obtained by using approximately 800 μCi of Tc-99m pertechnetate point source in a syringe. Remove the collimator from the detector head. Position the Tc-99m point source in front of the detector at a distance approximately 6 feet from the detector. For optimal imaging, the count rate should not be greater than 20,000 counts per second. Acquire an image for approximately 15,000K counts using a 64x64x16 matrix. Once the image is obtained, the image should be analyzed to ensure proper uniformity throughout the field of view.

Gamma camera resolution

Gamma camera resolution is the ability of the piece of equipment to diagnose or "*resolve*" lesions on a clinical nuclear medicine image. Resolution depends on the detector, the collimator, and all the camera electronics working as a unit to provide an accurate, diagnostic clinical image. In the nuclear medicine setting, as the distance of the patient from the detector increases, resolution decreases. Thus, to obtain optimal clinical nuclear medicine images, the patient should be positioned as close as possible to the detector head.

Evaluating procedures

Gamma camera resolution should be evaluated on a weekly basis in an intrinsic or extrinsic manner. A 4-quadrant bar phantom is required for the evaluation. For intrinsic resolution evaluation, remove the collimator and place the bar phantom directly on the crystal. For extrinsic evaluation, place the bar phantom directly on the collimator. The acquisition parameters are the same for both. Acquire a static image for approximately 5K counts on a 64x64x16 matrix. Once the image has been acquired, the image should be analyzed for adequate gamma camera resolution.

Center of rotation

Center of rotation is a term associated with SPECT imaging. A center of rotation evaluation is a quality control procedure to assess the mechanical alignment of the collimators, which enable the system to reconstruct from a center point during a circular SPECT acquisition. This evaluation is crucial to SPECT imaging because the center of rotation actually falls on a line that is fixed in space. The line is parallel to the imaging table and perpendicular to the plane of the gantry.

Evaluating procedures
For departments routinely performing SPECT imaging, center of rotation evaluations should be performed on a weekly basis, always in an extrinsic manner using an 800 μCi Tc-99m pertechnetate point source in a syringe. Place the Tc-99m point source slightly off center on the imaging table. Position the detector so the source is in the center of the field of view on both the anterior and lateral positions. Acquire a 360-degree SPECT image for 32 frames at 10 to 15

seconds per frame on a 64x64 matrix. If a dual head gamma camera is being used, this evaluation should be performed with the detectors in the 90- and 180-degree positions. The parameters are identical for both detector orientations. Once the acquisition is complete, the images should be analyzed to ensure proper collimator alignment.

Dead time

Dead time, also known as resolving time, is the interval immediately after an ionizing event. During this time, the Geiger-Mueller (GM) tube will not respond to any other ionizing events. Additional ionizing events that occur during this time will simply go unrecorded in the GM tube. Dead time in many GM tubes can be as high as 200 μsec.

Recombination region

In the recombination region, there is no voltage applied to the two electrodes, which means there is no direction given to ion pairs produced by the passing radiation. Without applied voltage, no ions are collected and no pulse is produced. Once voltage is applied, some ion pairs will be collected while others will recombine. As voltage increases, the collection of ion pairs will increase.

Ionization region

In the ionization region, the proportional increase in ion pair collection with increased voltage no longer exists. Instead, the curve flattens out and creates an area called a plateau. There is no increase in pulse height because the applied voltage is adequate to collect all ion pairs that are produced and there is no longer a chance of recombination in the ionization region.

Proportional region

In the proportional region, an increase in the number of ion pairs is once again seen. Whereas the voltage applied in the ionization region is sufficient to collect all ion pairs, the increased number of ion pairs in the proportional region is due to a phenomenon called gas amplification. The increased voltage applied through the proportional region adds energy to the ions that are being collected. This added energy allows the ions to ionize other particles in their paths. The additional ions will also be collected.

Non-proportional region

In the non-proportional region, voltage is once again increased and the relationship between applied voltage and collected ion pairs is no longer proportional. Instead, the pulse height is related more to the increase in applied voltage and less to the collected ion pairs.

Geiger-Mueller region

In the Geiger-Mueller region, the increase in applied voltage causes a sharp rise in the curve. The high voltage produces a high quantity or "*avalanche*" of ions making contact with the collecting electrode. This avalanche is due to the production of high-energy electrons and low-energy photons caused by bremsstrahlung. The high voltage in this region causes ionized particles to ionize other particles in their paths, causing the avalanche.

Continuous discharge region

In the continuous discharge region, voltage is once again increased and this once again causes the number of ion pairs collected to rise. This effect may be deceptive because it is primarily due to free electrons producing "*avalanches*" on the collecting electrode, not to ion pairs being collected. Continued operation in this region could cause the collecting electrodes to be damaged or destroyed.

Scatter radiation

Scatter radiation is radiation that is diverted from its path due to some kind of collision. In a clinical nuclear medicine setting, full-energy photons emitted directly toward the detector are normally counted and included in the data used to form the image. However, scatter radiation may also make its way to the detector and be counted, even though it is lower in energy and should be differentiated from full-energy photons. Scatter radiation, if accepted, will increase the count rate and degrade image quality.

Radiation absorption

Radiation absorption is the total dissipation of radioactive energy into the absorbing material. Radiation that is absorbed never reaches the detector and is not included in count-rate statistics. Radiation absorption can occur in three different sites: the source itself, the media between the radioactive source and the detector, and the detector itself. Regardless of the site, absorption affects the count rate in the same manner by reducing the number of radioactive photons reaching the detector.

ICANL

The Intersocietal Commission for the Accreditation of Nuclear Medicine Laboratories (ICANL) is an accrediting body that imposes standards for nuclear cardiology, nuclear medicine, and PET facilities that must be met for accreditation. Accreditation is extremely important because many insurance reimbursements are based on procedures being performed at accredited facilities.

Facilities that are not accredited may not be reimbursed for procedures performed at those facilities.

ACR

The American College of Radiology (ACR) is an accrediting body that imposes standards for nuclear cardiology, nuclear medicine, PET facilities, and all other imaging modalities such as CT and MRI. ACR standards must be met to obtain accreditation. Accreditation is extremely important for imaging facilities because many insurance reimbursements are based on procedures being performed at accredited facilities. Facilities that are not accredited may not be reimbursed for procedures performed at those facilities.

MIPPA law

The Medicare Improvements for Patients and Providers Act (MIPPA) is a piece of 2008 legislation that requires all non-hospital centers of advanced diagnostic imaging to obtain accreditation from the American College of Radiology (ACR) or the Intersocietal Commission for the Accreditation of Nuclear Medicine Laboratories (ICANL) by January 2012. This law does not only apply to nuclear medicine facilities. It applies to all forms of advanced diagnostic imaging, such as CT and MRI.

Radiation worker pregnancy declaration

A female radiation worker has the right to declare a pregnancy at any time during the pregnancy. If she chooses not to declare the pregnancy, no measures need to be taken and the facility is not responsible for the safety of the fetus. If she declares the pregnancy, she must do so in writing and include the approximate date of impregnation. In addition, a fetal badge must be issued and worn in the abdominal region to quantify radiation exposure to the fetus, which must not exceed 500 mrem for the total duration of the pregnancy.

Quality management program

A quality management program is of great importance for facilities that perform radioactive therapeutic procedures. The purpose of a quality management program is to reduce the risk of administration errors and reportable events. There are 5 main objectives essential to any quality management program:

- A written directive is obtained prior to administration of any radioactive material
- The patient is verified with more than one method
- All calculations and courses of treatment follow the written directive
- The radioactive material is administered according to the written directive
- Appropriate action is taken if deviation from the written directive occurs

Written directive

A written directive is needed when administering any therapeutic dose of radioactive material. A written directive is not required when administering radioactive materials for diagnostic purposes. Prior to administering a therapeutic dose, a written directive must be obtained and it must contain the following information.

- The patient's name
- The name, dose, and route of administration of the radioactive material
- The purpose for the administration of radioactive materials

- The date and time of the administration of radioactive materials
- The signature of the authorized user performing or overseeing the administration of radioactive material
-

Department records retained for 3 years

All records of department wipe tests and surveys; all dose calibrator evaluations such as linearity, constancy, and accuracy; all records of patient dose administrations, both diagnostic and therapeutic; all written directives; all records of radioactive trash decayed and disposed of; receipts for all radioactive shipments.

Department records retained for 5 years

All records of radioactive materials transferred from one facility to another; the department inventory of all sealed sources including flood sources, radioactive markers, and attenuation correction sources; all leak tests that have been performed on the inventory of sealed sources; records of all administration errors.

Department records retained indefinitely

All records of personnel radiation exposure; all minutes from radiation safety committee meetings (these are kept indefinitely or for the duration of the radioactive materials license); dose calibrator geometry evaluations (these are kept indefinitely or for the life of the dose calibrator); all records of I-131 bioassays performed on radiation workers.

Bioassay

A bioassay should be performed on all radiation workers involved in I-131 therapeutic procedures. A bioassay ensures that the thyroid is not being over-exposed to I-131. This is primarily a concern when I-131 is administered in liquid form. There is very little risk of thyroid exposure when it is administered in capsule form. Bioassay results need to be retained indefinitely. If a radiation worker has absorbed more than 3 µCi of I-131 in a year, the worker should be relieved of isotope handling duties for the remainder of the year.

License code 10 CFR 35.100

License code 10 CFR 35.100 allows the use of unsealed byproduct material for uptake, dilution, and excretion studies in which a written directive is not required. This code primarily permits the use of radioactive materials for laboratory tests in which radioactive materials are injected, inhaled, or ingested and then a bodily fluid such as blood or urine is tested for radionuclide uptake. Examples of procedures governed by code 10 CFR 35.100 include ^{51}Cr chromate for red cell survival and red cell mass studies, ^{57}Co for vitamin B-12 absorption studies, and ^{59}Fe citrate for iron absorption, iron plasma clearance and turnover, and iron red blood cell uptake studies. Code 10 CFR 35.100 also requires nuclear medicine facilities to have a survey meter capable of detecting dose rates from 0.1 to 100 mR/hr.

License code 10 CFR 35.200

Code 10 CFR 35.200 allows the use of unsealed byproduct material for imaging and localization studies in which a written directive is not required. This code governs imaging procedures that require a photon emitter with energy sufficient to be imaged, primarily with a gamma camera. Localization studies are imaging studies in which localized radioactive material is detected by a radiation probe. Although the use of Tc-99m for imaging studies is the primary focus of Code 10 CFR 35.200, this code governs all other isotopes used in nuclear medicine, such as I-131 and TI-201.

License code 10 CFR 35.300

License code 10 CFR 35.300 allows the use any unsealed byproduct material that is prepared for medical purposes and requires a written directive. This code governs all radioactive materials that are administered for therapeutic purposes, such as I-131, Sm-153, and Y-90. It states that the radioactive material must be obtained from a licensed manufacturer, prepared by a licensed nuclear pharmacist, and administered by an authorized user or individual supervised by an authorized user.

License code 10 CFR 35.400

License code 10 CFR 35.400 allows the use of radioactive material for brachytherapeutic purposes. Isotopes covered under Code CFR 35.400 are Cs-137 for topical, interstitial, or intracavitary treatment, Co-60 for topical, interstitial, or intracavitary treatment, Gold (Au-198) seeds for interstitial treatment, Ir-192 for interstitial treatment, Sr-90 eye applicators, I-125 seeds for interstitial treatment, and Pd-103 seeds for interstitial treatment.

License code 10 CFR 35.500

License code 10 CFR 35.500 permits the use of sealed sources for diagnostic purposes. Examples of radioactive materials governed under this code are I-125, Am-241, and Ga-153 as sealed sources in devices for bone mineral

analysis. I-125 is also used as a sealed source in portable imaging devices. Sealed sources and devices should have certificates of authorization for diagnostic use on file in the National Sealed Source and Device Registry.

License code 10 CFR 35.600

License code 10 CFR 35.600 permits the use of a sealed source in a remote afterloader unit, teletherapy unit, or gamma stereotactic radiosurgery unit. This code primarily regulates the use of Co-60 and Cs-137 in teletherapy units. The isotopes should have certificates of authorization on file in the National Sealed Source and Device Registry. Code 10 CFR 35.600 also governs isotopes used for research in accordance with an active Investigational Device Exemption (IDE) accepted by the FDA.

Radiation Brachytherapy

Brachytherapy is a type of radiation therapy in which the radioactive source is surgically implanted into a patient. Brachytherapy is also referred to as internal radiotherapy, sealed source radiotherapy, curietherapy, or endocurietherapy. Brachytherapy is commonly used for the treatment of prostate, breast, cervical, and skin cancers. Brachytherapy can be performed alone or in conjunction with other therapeutic forms such as chemotherapy.

NRC occupational radiation exposure limits

For adult radiation workers, the total effective dose equivalent should not exceed 5 rem per calendar year. The total organ dose equivalent should not exceed 50 rem per calendar year. The total organ dose equivalent includes exposure to all organs of the body except the lens of the eye. The external dose of radiation to the lenses of the eyes should not exceed 15 rem per calendar year. The dose to the skin or any extremity should not exceed 50 rem per calendar year. For minor employees, the exposure limits are 10% of those for adult employees.

RSO

All facilities that maintain a radioactive materials license must appoint an RSO (radiation safety officer) who is responsible for the safe use of radiation and radioactive materials. The RSO is also responsible for recommending or approving corrective actions, identifying radiation safety problems, initiating action, and ensuring compliance with regulations. Other duties of the RSO include annual review of the radiation safety program for adherence to ALARA (as low as reasonably achievable) concepts, quarterly review of external and occupational exposures of authorized users and workers to determine that their exposures are ALARA, and quarterly review of records of radiation level surveys. In addition, the RSO reviews radiation levels in unrestricted and restricted areas to determine that they were ALARA during the previous quarter.

RSC

All facilities that perform more than 2 advanced imaging modalities are required to have an RSC (radiation safety committee) responsible for the safe use of radiation and radioactive materials. The committee must consist of a radiation safety officer, a member of the facility's administration, an authorized user, and a member of each department in which radioactive materials are used.

Diagnostic and Therapeutic Procedures

Opioid medications

Morphine and other opioid medications such as hydromorphone cause contraction of the Sphincter of Oddi and common bile duct, resulting in delayed emptying of bile through the common bile duct. In addition, morphine and hydromorphone may cause bile to fill the gallbladder by increasing the pressure of the Sphincter of Oddi, leading to a false-negative result for acute cholecystitis.

Regadenoson in pharmaceutical stress testing

Regadenoson is the newest drug approved for pharmaceutical stress testing. It activates the A2A adenosine receptor to produce coronary dilation and increase blood flow through the coronary vessels. The only contraindication to regadenoson for pharmaceutical stress testing is the presence of second or third-degree AV block, unless the patient has a pacemaker. Regadenoson is generally better tolerated than other commonly used drugs for pharmaceutical stress testing such as adenosine and dobutamine. Maximum absorption of regadenoson occurs 1 to 4 minutes after administration. Therefore, the isotope should be administered approximately 1 minute after regadenoson.

Bexxar

Bexxar is an I-131-labeled monoclonal antibody treatment for follicular, non-Hodgkin lymphoma that has recurred after chemotherapy. The I-131-labeled monoclonal antibody attaches to a protein found only on the surface of B lymphocytes such as the cancerous B-cells found in many forms of non-

Hodgkin's lymphoma. The radioactivity targets and destroys the B-cell. Bexxar is given as an intravenous injection once a week for 2 weeks. The first dose is given with just a small amount of I-131. This first infusion is called the dosimetric dose. Since I-131 is both a gamma and beta radiation emitter, it can be imaged directly because the imaging cameras detect gamma radiation only. (The beta radiation is what actually kills the lymphoma, however.) Approximately 2 to 4 days after the dosimetric dose and again at approximately 6 to 7 days after, the patient is scanned to see where the Bexxar is being distributed in the body. The therapeutic dose is given between 7 and 14 days after the dosimetric dose, once the optimum dose is calculated based on the previous scans.

Zevalin

Zevalin is a Y-90-labeled monoclonal antibody treatment for follicular non-Hodgkin lymphoma that has not been treated or has recurred after chemotherapy. A Zevalin therapeutic regimen consists of the monoclonal antibody rituximab, In-111-labeled Zevalin for imaging, and Y-90-labeled Zevalin for therapy.

Zevalin therapeutic regimen

A Zevalin therapeutic regimen is a 3-stage process that can take from 7 to 9 days to complete.
Day One:
- The patient should be premedicated with acetaminophen and diphenhydramine followed by intravenous administration of rituximab. Within 4 hours of rituximab infusion, In-111-labeled Zevalin is given as an intravenous injection

Day Three or Four:
- An imaging scan is done to confirm acceptable distribution of In-111-labeled Zevalin throughout the patient's body and to ensure it is safe for the patient to receive the therapeutic dose of Y-90-labeled Zevalin

Day Seven, Eight, or Nine:
- Once again, the patient should be premedicated with acetaminophen and diphenhydramine followed by administration of a rituximab infusion. Within 4 hours of the rituximab infusion, Y-90-labeled Zevalin is given as an intravenous injection. The Y-90-labeled Zevalin is a monoclonal antibody combined with a radioisotope that attacks B-cells and provides the therapeutic component of the Zevalin regimen

Metastron

Metastron is radioactive, beta-emitting Sr-89 used to treat the pain associated with widespread metastatic lesions in the bone. The beta particles emitted from Sr-89 have a maximum energy of 1.46 MeV. Metastron is administered via slow intravenous injection with an activity of 4 mCi. It should be noted that Metastron therapy does not instantly relieve the pain, but may take up to 7 days to do so. In fact, pain may even get worse or "flare up" a day or two post-injection. Another side effect of Metastron is low blood count. If additional doses of Metastron are required, 90 days should elapse between doses.

Quadramet

Quadramet is a radioactive material used to treat the pain associated with widespread metastatic lesions in the bone. Quadramet is commonly used in patients that have osteoblastic metastatic bone lesions confirmed by a whole body bone scan. Sm-153 emits both beta particles and gamma rays. The energy of the beta particles ranges from 640 to 810keV. The gamma ray energy is 103 keV. It is possible to perform a whole body scan using the 103 keV gamma ray. The activity of Quadramet is 1 mCi/kg. It should be noted that Quadramet therapy does not instantly relieve the pain, but may take up to 7 days to do so. In fact, pain may even get worse or "flare up" a day or two post-injection.

Uniformity procedure performed on PET scanners daily for quality control

The uniformity check, also referred to as a sinogram check, is a quality control procedure that should be performed on PET scanners daily. Uniformity is evaluated using either a Ge-68 or Cs-137 source. The radioactive source is mounted in brackets on the gantry of the PET camera and rotated around the scan field so each detector is equally exposed to the radioactive source. If all detectors are functioning properly, there will be a homogeneous response from all detectors and a uniform sinogram will result. If a detector pair is malfunctioning, a streak will occur in the sinogram.

Daily sinogram check

The daily sinogram should be compared to the sinogram that was performed during acceptance testing of the PET camera. The difference between the two sinograms is expressed by a value known as the average variance, which is an indicator of various detector problems. If the average variance exceeds 2.5, then efforts should be made to recalibrate the PET scanner. If the average variance exceeds 5.0, then the manufacturer

should be called to service the machine immediately.

Normalization procedure performed on PET scanners weekly for quality control

The normalization procedure should be performed on PET scanners on a weekly basis to correct for non-uniformities that occur in PET images. The procedure requires a 20-cm rod source containing 1 to 3 mCi of Ge-68, which is placed in the center of the field of view. All detectors are equally exposed to the Ge-68 rod source, and the resulting data are used to produce correction factors for each detector. To ensure better accuracy in normalization, long acquisitions such as 6 to 8 hours or even overnight are recommended.

CT number

The CT number represents the attenuation properties of body tissues in each pixel on the Hounsfield scale, which ranks various materials by their attenuation properties. On the Hounsfield scale, water is a reference point with a value of 0. Air is another reference point with a value of -100. Most soft tissues encountered in CT scanning have values ranging from 30 to 60, whereas dense bone has a value of 1,000. CT numbers over 100 generally represent calcification.

Coincidence timing calibration performed on PET Scanners

The coincidence timing calibration is a critical evaluation of PET scanners that detects and corrects timing differences in the detectors of the scanner. The test is usually performed by placing a positron source between the detector rings and recording the time differences (coincidence events) between the signals. Since positrons travel at 180 degrees from each other at identical speeds, they should hit the detectors simultaneously. If they do not, it means there is malfunctioning of the detectors, photomultiplier tubes, or electronic circuitry.

Photomultiplier tube

A photomultiplier tube is a light-sensitive device that usually contains one photocathode and a series of 10 dynodes. The photomultiplier tube is optically connected to the sodium iodide crystal in gamma cameras. The purpose of the photomultiplier tube is to convert the light energy from the crystal to electrical energy and amplify the resulting pulse of electricity. The resulting pulse height is equally proportional to the energy of the gamma ray coming into contact with the sodium iodide crystal.

PACS

PACS stands for Picture Archiving and Communication Systems. PACS has greatly benefitted the field of medical imaging by eliminating the need for films; all patient images can now be kept electronically. PACS has four major benefits:

- Eliminates the need for films, thus reducing costs and space requirements for storage of medical images
- Allows for rapid retrieval of all medical images performed on a patient
- Access to images that were acquired with multiple modalities
- Simultaneous access to images performed at multiple sites

PACS and Radiology Information Systems (RIS) work simultaneously to support the entire function of the radiology department.

RIS

RIS is an acronym for Radiology Information Systems, which are computerized databases used primarily for storage, manipulation, and distribution of patient radiological data and images. RIS systems commonly support patient scheduling and registration, request and document scanning, faxing and e-mailing of patient exam results, and radiology workflow management. RIS and PACS work simultaneously to support the entire radiology department.

Filtered back projection

Filtered back projection is the most commonly used technique for image reconstruction. The use of filters is an easy and effective way to remove the star pattern around each photon. Filtered back projection is the most effective technique to reconstruct tomographic acquisitions because the resulting images are enhanced.

Iterative technique for tomographic image reconstruction

The iterative technique for image reconstruction, sometimes referred to as the algebraic technique, was one of the first image reconstruction techniques applied to nuclear medicine. For many years, it had largely been replaced by filtered techniques. But with the emergence of attenuation correction, it has come back to the forefront of the image reconstruction field. The iterative technique is commonly used when reconstructing SPECT images that have been corrected for attenuation. The iterative method for reconstruction ensures the true number of counts in each pixel.

Ramp filter

The ramp filter provides the highest level of image resolution but also generates the greatest amount of noise. If a ramp filter is chosen for nuclear medicine image reconstruction, the resulting images may contain sharp areas of contrast and possibly ring artifacts. In order for the ramp filter to be an effective tool, it should be used on images that have extremely high count rates. The ramp filter is generally of no use in the clinical nuclear medicine setting.

Parzen filter

The Parzen filter produces the exact opposite effect of the ramp filter. It provides the lowest level of image resolution but also generates the least amount of noise. If the Parzen filter is chosen for nuclear medicine image reconstruction, the resulting images may appear excessively smooth, even to the extent of masking lesions. The use of a Parzen filter for SPECT reconstruction is generally counterproductive because it may mask lesions.

Hamming filter

The Hamming filter is the best filter for reconstructing SPECT studies that have a generally low number of counts. The Hamming filter is the proper choice for reconstructing images acquired with Tl-201, Ga-67, or bone SPECT scans. The Hamming filter smoothes out any imperfections and reduces any noise caused by lack of data. The Hamming filter permits a diagnostic-quality image even if the count rate is excessively low.

Butterworth filter

The Butterworth filter is by far the most used filter in nuclear medicine, particularly for cardiac, brain, and liver SPECT imaging, because it provides the best compromise between smoothness and sharpness. The Butterworth filter is also the most versatile filter in that it allows an additional adjustment to ensure the highest quality image. Whereas all SPECT filters can be adjusted using a parameter called cutoff frequency, an additional parameter known as order is available with the Butterworth filter.

SPECT processing filters cutoff frequency

The cutoff frequency specifies the bandwidth of the filter and determines which data is accepted and which is eliminated from the image. The lower the cutoff frequency, the more the image can be influenced by scatter or incompletely absorbed photons, therefore, the lower the cutoff frequency, the lower the resolution and the smoother the image, he higher the cutoff frequency, the greater the image resolution.

Butterworth filters

The Butterworth filter is the only filter in nuclear medicine that can be further modified. This is accomplished with the parameter of order, which modifies the Butterworth filter by allowing the slope of filter function to be altered. This type of alteration allows for the greatest compromise between the smoothness of the image and the sharpness of the edge of the image. The parameter of order allows the nuclear medicine technologist to provide the highest quality images to ensure accurate diagnoses.

Patient Care and Education

Weekly quality control procedures

Department surveys should be performed in all areas where radioactive materials are used and stored. A department wipe test should be performed in all areas where radioactive materials are used and stored. Bar phantom flood images should be performed on all gamma cameras to ensure proper resolution. Center of rotation acquisitions should be performed on all gamma cameras in which SPECT imaging is acquired.

Informed consent

Informed consent is communication between a patient and a healthcare provider that results in the patient giving the provider permission to perform a specific medical procedure. Informed consent means the patient has received comprehensive information about his or her diagnosis, the procedure to be performed, the risks of the procedure, alternatives to the procedure and their risks and the risks of not having the treatment or procedure. As part of informed consent, the patient should be permitted to ask questions to gain a thorough understanding of the recommended treatment. Informed consent is an ethical obligation and legal requirement in all 50 states.

HIPAA

HIPAA is the Health Insurance Portability and Accountability Act approved by congress and signed into law in 1996. HIPAA was enacted to protect the privacy of personal health information by setting limits on the use and disclosure of such information without patient authorization. The Act also gives patients rights over their health information, including the right to examine and obtain copies of their health records and the right to request corrections.

Living will

A living will is one form of advance health care directive. It spells out a patient's wishes regarding medical care should he or she be incapable of making those decisions when a medical situation arises. A living will also empowers another individual to make medical decisions on the patient's behalf.

Medical and surgical asepsis

Medical asepsis is the technique used to prevent the spread of microorganisms. Surgical asepsis is a technique or procedure to eliminate all microorganisms from an object, instrument or area. Medical asepsis means clean. Surgical asepsis means sterile.

Bloodborne pathogen

Bloodborne pathogens are microorganisms in the blood or other body fluids that can cause illness and disease in people. These microorganisms can be transmitted through contact with contaminated blood and body fluids. The majority of the population immediately refers to the HIV virus or AIDS when defining bloodborne pathogens. However, hepatitis B and C are much more common in the medical setting.

Bloodborne pathogens exposure

A medical professional can be exposed to bloodborne pathogens by accidental puncture wounds from needles, scalpels, broken glass or razor blades. An individual can also be exposed if contaminated body fluids come into contact with an open wound on the skin. The hepatitis B virus can actually be transmitted indirectly when medical professional touches dried or caked-on blood and then touches the eyes, nose, or mouth.

Universal precautions

Universal precautions are medical practice guidelines used to avoid contact with a patient's blood or bodily fluids. Healthcare workers adhere to universal precautions by wearing nonporous garments such as gowns, gloves, goggles, and face shields whenever contact with bodily fluids can occur. Universal precautions should always be used when there is a risk of exposure to blood, semen, vaginal secretions, or cerebrospinal fluid, but they are not required to prevent contact with feces, vomit, sputum, sweat, or urine.

Nosocomial infection

Nosocomial infections, also known as hospital-acquired infections, are infections directly related to treatment in a hospital or other healthcare facility. Nosocomial infections are commonly caused by healthcare practitioners not performing proper hygiene such as hand washing. These infections are also commonly passed on by healthcare practitioners simply moving from patient to patient during the work day. The use of universal precautions and proper sanitation protocols should limit the occurrence of nosocomial infections.

Special Report: What Your Test Score Will Tell You About Your IQ

Did you know that most standardized tests correlate very strongly with IQ? In fact, your general intelligence is a better predictor of your success than any other factor, and most tests intentionally measure this trait to some degree to ensure that those selected by the test are truly qualified for the test's purposes.

Before we can delve into the relation between your test score and IQ, I will first have to explain what exactly is IQ. Here's the formula:

Your IQ = 100 + (Number of standard deviations below or above the average)*15

Now, let's define standard deviations by using an example. If we have 5 people with 5 different heights, then first we calculate the average. Let's say the average was 65 inches. The standard deviation is the "average distance" away from the average of each of the members. It is a direct measure of variability - if the 5 people included Jackie Chan and Shaquille O'Neal, obviously there's a lot more variability in that group than a group of 5 sisters who are all within 6 inches in height of each other. The standard deviation uses a number to characterize the average range of difference within a group.

A convenient feature of most groups is that they have a "normal" distribution- makes sense that most things would be normal, right? Without getting into a bunch of statistical mumbo-jumbo, you just need to know that if you know the average of the group and the standard deviation, you can successfully predict someone's percentile rank in the group.

Confused? Let me give you an example. If instead of 5 people's heights, we had 100 people, we could figure out their rank in height JUST by knowing the average, standard deviation, and their height. We wouldn't need to know each person's height and manually rank them; we could just predict their rank based on three numbers.

What this means is that you can take your PERCENTILE rank that is often given with your test and relate this to your RELATIVE IQ of people taking the test - that is, your IQ relative to the people taking the test. Obviously, there's no way to know your actual IQ because the people taking a standardized test are usually not very good samples of the general population- many of those with extremely low IQ's never achieve a level of success or competency necessary to complete a typical standardized test. In fact, professional psychologists who measure IQ actually have to use non-written tests that can fairly measure the IQ of those not able to complete a traditional test.

The bottom line is to not take your test score too seriously, but it is fun to compute your "relative IQ" among the people who took the test with you. I've done the calculations below. Just look up your percentile rank in the left and then you'll see your "relative IQ" for your test in the right hand column.

Percentile Rank	Your Relative IQ		Percentile Rank	Your Relative IQ
99	135		59	103
98	131		58	103
97	128		57	103
96	126		56	102
95	125		55	102
94	123		54	102
93	122		53	101
92	121		52	101
91	120		51	100
90	119		50	100
89	118		49	100
88	118		48	99
87	117		47	99
86	116		46	98
85	116		45	98
84	115		44	98
83	114		43	97
82	114		42	97
81	113		41	97
80	113		40	96
79	112		39	96
78	112		38	95
77	111		37	95
76	111		36	95
75	110		35	94
74	110		34	94
73	109		33	93
72	109		32	93
71	108		31	93
70	108		30	92
69	107		29	92
68	107		28	91
67	107		27	91
66	106		26	90
65	106		25	90
64	105		24	89
63	105		23	89
62	105		22	88
61	104		21	88
60	104		20	87

Special Report: What is Test Anxiety and How to Overcome It?

The very nature of tests caters to some level of anxiety, nervousness or tension, just as we feel for any important event that occurs in our lives. A little bit of anxiety or nervousness can be a good thing. It helps us with motivation, and makes achievement just that much sweeter. However, too much anxiety can be a problem; especially if it hinders our ability to function and perform.

"Test anxiety," is the term that refers to the emotional reactions that some test-takers experience when faced with a test or exam. Having a fear of testing and exams is based upon a rational fear, since the test-taker's performance can shape the course of an academic career. Nevertheless, experiencing excessive fear of examinations will only interfere with the test-takers ability to perform and his/her chances to be successful.

There are a large variety of causes that can contribute to the development and sensation of test anxiety. These include, but are not limited to lack of performance and worrying about issues surrounding the test.

Lack of Preparation

Lack of preparation can be identified by the following behaviors or situations:

Not scheduling enough time to study, and therefore cramming the night before the test or exam
Managing time poorly, to create the sensation that there is not enough time to do everything
Failing to organize the text information in advance, so that the study material consists of the entire text and not simply the pertinent information
Poor overall studying habits

Worrying, on the other hand, can be related to both the test taker, and many other factors around him/her that will be affected by the results of the test. These include worrying about:

Previous performances on similar exams, or exams in general
How friends and other students are achieving
The negative consequences that will result from a poor grade or failure

There are three primary elements to test anxiety. Physical components which involve the same typical bodily reactions as those to acute anxiety (to be discussed below).

Emotional factors have to do with fear or panic. Mental or cognitive issues concerning attention spans and memory abilities.

Physical Signals

There are many different symptoms of test anxiety, and these are not limited to mental and emotional strain. Frequently there are a range of physical signals that will let a test taker know that he/she is suffering from test anxiety. These bodily changes can include the following:

Perspiring
Sweaty palms
Wet, trembling hands
Nausea
Dry mouth
A knot in the stomach
Headache
Faintness
Muscle tension
Aching shoulders, back and neck
Rapid heart beat
Feeling too hot/cold

To recognize the sensation of test anxiety, a test-taker should monitor him/herself for the following sensations:

The physical distress symptoms as listed above
Emotional sensitivity, expressing emotional feelings such as the need to cry or laugh too much, or a sensation of anger or helplessness
A decreased ability to think, causing the test-taker to blank out or have racing thoughts that are hard to organize or control.

Though most students will feel some level of anxiety when faced with a test or exam, the majority can cope with that anxiety and maintain it at a manageable level. However, those who cannot are faced with a very real and very serious condition, which can and should be controlled for the immeasurable benefit of this sufferer.

Naturally, these sensations lead to negative results for the testing experience. The most common effects of test anxiety have to do with nervousness and mental blocking.

Nervousness

Nervousness can appear in several different levels:

The test-taker's difficulty, or even inability to read and understand the questions on the test
The difficulty or inability to organize thoughts to a coherent form
The difficulty or inability to recall key words and concepts relating to the testing questions (especially essays)
The receipt of poor grades on a test, though the test material was well known by the test taker

Conversely, a person may also experience mental blocking, which involves:

Blanking out on test questions
Only remembering the correct answers to the questions when the test has already finished.

Fortunately for test anxiety sufferers, beating these feelings, to a large degree, has to do with proper preparation. When a test taker has a feeling of preparedness, then anxiety will be dramatically lessened.

The first step to resolving anxiety issues is to distinguish which of the two types of anxiety are being suffered. If the anxiety is a direct result of a lack of preparation, this should be considered a normal reaction, and the anxiety level (as opposed to the test results) shouldn't be anything to worry about. However, if, when adequately prepared, the test-taker still panics, blanks out, or seems to overreact, this is not a fully rational reaction. While this can be considered normal too, there are many ways to combat and overcome these effects.

Remember that anxiety cannot be entirely eliminated, however, there are ways to minimize it, to make the anxiety easier to manage. Preparation is one of the best ways to minimize test anxiety. Therefore the following techniques are wise in order to best fight off any anxiety that may want to build.

To begin with, try to avoid cramming before a test, whenever it is possible. By trying to memorize an entire term's worth of information in one day, you'll be shocking your system, and not giving yourself a very good chance to absorb the information. This is an easy path to anxiety, so for those who suffer from test anxiety, cramming should not even be considered an option.

Instead of cramming, work throughout the semester to combine all of the material which is presented throughout the semester, and work on it gradually as the course goes by, making sure to master the main concepts first, leaving minor details for a week or so before the test.

To study for the upcoming exam, be sure to pose questions that may be on the examination, to gauge the ability to answer them by integrating the ideas from your texts, notes and lectures, as well as any supplementary readings.

If it is truly impossible to cover all of the information that was covered in that particular term, concentrate on the most important portions that can be covered very well. Learn these concepts as best as possible, so that when the test comes, a goal can be made to use these concepts as presentations of your knowledge.

In addition to study habits, changes in attitude are critical to beating a struggle with test anxiety. In fact, an improvement of the perspective over the entire test-taking experience can actually help a test taker to enjoy studying and therefore improve the overall experience. Be certain not to overemphasize the significance of the grade - know that the result of the test is neither a reflection of self worth, nor is it a measure of intelligence; one grade will not predict a person's future success.

To improve an overall testing outlook, the following steps should be tried:

Keeping in mind that the most reasonable expectation for taking a test is to expect to try to demonstrate as much of what you know as you possibly can.
Reminding ourselves that a test is only one test; this is not the only one, and there will be others.
The thought of thinking of oneself in an irrational, all-or-nothing term should be avoided at all costs.
A reward should be designated for after the test, so there's something to look forward to. Whether it is going to a movie, going out to eat, or simply visiting friends, schedule it in advance, and do it no matter what result is expected on the exam.

Test-takers should also keep in mind that the basics are some of the most important things, even beyond anti-anxiety techniques and studying. Never neglect the basic social, emotional and biological needs, in order to try to absorb information. In order to best achieve, these three factors must be held as just as important as the studying itself.

Study Steps

Remember the following important steps for studying:

Maintain healthy nutrition and exercise habits. Continue both your recreational activities and social pass times. These both contribute to your physical and emotional well being.
Be certain to get a good amount of sleep, especially the night before the test, because when you're overtired you are not able to perform to the best of your best ability.
Keep the studying pace to a moderate level by taking breaks when they are needed, and varying the work whenever possible, to keep the mind fresh instead of getting bored.

When enough studying has been done that all the material that can be learned has been learned, and the test taker is prepared for the test, stop studying and do something relaxing such as listening to music, watching a movie, or taking a warm bubble bath.

There are also many other techniques to minimize the uneasiness or apprehension that is experienced along with test anxiety before, during, or even after the examination. In fact, there are a great deal of things that can be done to stop anxiety from interfering with lifestyle and performance. Again, remember that anxiety will not be eliminated entirely, and it shouldn't be. Otherwise that "up" feeling for exams would not exist, and most of us depend on that sensation to perform better than usual. However, this anxiety has to be at a level that is manageable.

Of course, as we have just discussed, being prepared for the exam is half the battle right away. Attending all classes, finding out what knowledge will be expected on the exam, and knowing the exam schedules are easy steps to lowering anxiety. Keeping up with work will remove the need to cram, and efficient study habits will eliminate wasted time. Studying should be done in an ideal location for concentration, so that it is simple to become interested in the material and give it complete attention. A method such as SQ3R (Survey, Question, Read, Recite, Review) is a wonderful key to follow to make sure that the study habits are as effective as possible, especially in the case of learning from a textbook. Flashcards are great techniques for memorization. Learning to take good notes will mean that notes will be full of useful information, so that less sifting will need to be done to seek out what is pertinent for studying. Reviewing notes after class and then again on occasion will keep the information fresh in the mind. From notes that have been taken summary sheets and outlines can be made for simpler reviewing.

A study group can also be a very motivational and helpful place to study, as there will be a sharing of ideas, all of the minds can work together, to make sure that everyone understands, and the studying will be made more interesting because it will be a social occasion.

Basically, though, as long as the test-taker remains organized and self confident, with efficient study habits, less time will need to be spent studying, and higher grades will be achieved.

To become self confident, there are many useful steps. The first of these is "self talk." It has been shown through extensive research, that self-talk for students who suffer from test anxiety, should be well monitored, in order to make sure that it contributes to self confidence as opposed to sinking the student. Frequently the self talk of test-anxious students is negative or self-defeating, thinking that everyone else is smarter and faster, that they always mess up, and that if they don't do well, they'll fail the entire course. It is important to decreasing anxiety that awareness is made of self talk. Try writing any negative self thoughts and then disputing them with a positive statement instead. Begin self-encouragement as though it was a friend speaking. Repeat positive statements to help reprogram the mind to believing in successes instead of failures.

Helpful Techniques

Other extremely helpful techniques include:

Self-visualization of doing well and reaching goals
While aiming for an "A" level of understanding, don't try to "overprotect" by setting your expectations lower. This will only convince the mind to stop studying in order to meet the lower expectations.
Don't make comparisons with the results or habits of other students. These are individual factors, and different things work for different people, causing different results.
Strive to become an expert in learning what works well, and what can be done in order to improve. Consider collecting this data in a journal.
Create rewards for after studying instead of doing things before studying that will only turn into avoidance behaviors.
Make a practice of relaxing - by using methods such as progressive relaxation, self-hypnosis, guided imagery, etc - in order to make relaxation an automatic sensation.
Work on creating a state of relaxed concentration so that concentrating will take on the focus of the mind, so that none will be wasted on worrying.
Take good care of the physical self by eating well and getting enough sleep.
Plan in time for exercise and stick to this plan.

Beyond these techniques, there are other methods to be used before, during and after the test that will help the test-taker perform well in addition to overcoming anxiety.

Before the exam comes the academic preparation. This involves establishing a study schedule and beginning at least one week before the actual date of the test. By doing this, the anxiety of not having enough time to study for the test will be automatically eliminated. Moreover, this will make the studying a much more effective experience, ensuring that the learning will be an easier process. This relieves much undue pressure on the test-taker.

Summary sheets, note cards, and flash cards with the main concepts and examples of these main concepts should be prepared in advance of the actual studying time. A topic should never be eliminated from this process. By omitting a topic because it isn't expected to be on the test is only setting up the test-taker for anxiety should it actually appear on the exam. Utilize the course syllabus for laying out the topics that should be studied. Carefully go over the notes that were made in class, paying special attention to any of the issues that the professor took special care to emphasize while lecturing in class. In the textbooks, use the chapter review, or if possible, the chapter tests, to begin your review.

It may even be possible to ask the instructor what information will be covered on the exam, or what the format of the exam will be (for example, multiple choice, essay, free form, true-false). Additionally, see if it is possible to find out how many questions will be on the test. If a review sheet or sample test has been offered by the professor, make good use of it, above anything else, for the preparation for the test. Another great resource for getting to know the examination is reviewing tests from previous semesters. Use these tests to review, and aim to achieve a 100% score on each of the possible topics. With a few exceptions, the goal that you set for yourself is the highest one that you will reach.

Take all of the questions that were assigned as homework, and rework them to any other possible course material. The more problems reworked, the more skill and confidence will form as a result. When forming the solution to a problem, write out each of the steps. Don't simply do head work. By doing as many steps on paper as possible, much clarification and therefore confidence will be formed. Do this with as many homework problems as possible, before checking the answers. By checking the answer after each problem, reinforcement will exist, that will not be on the exam. Study situations should be as exam-like as possible, to prime the test-taker's system for the experience. By waiting to check the answers at the end, a psychological advantage will be formed, to decrease the stress factor.

Another fantastic reason for not cramming is the avoidance of confusion in concepts, especially when it comes to mathematics. 8-10 hours of study will become one hundred percent more effective if it is spread out over a week or at least several days, instead of doing it all in one sitting. Recognize that the human brain requires time in order to assimilate new material, so frequent breaks and a span of study time over several days will be much more beneficial.

Additionally, don't study right up until the point of the exam. Studying should stop a minimum of one hour before the exam begins. This allows the brain to rest and put things in their proper order. This will also provide the time to become as relaxed as possible when going into the examination room. The test-taker will also have time to eat well and eat sensibly. Know that the brain needs food as much as the rest of the body. With enough food and enough sleep, as well as a relaxed attitude, the body and the mind are primed for success.

Avoid any anxious classmates who are talking about the exam. These students only spread anxiety, and are not worth sharing the anxious sentimentalities.

Before the test also involves creating a positive attitude, so mental preparation should also be a point of concentration. There are many keys to creating a positive attitude. Should fears become rushing in, make a visualization of taking the exam, doing well, and seeing an A written on the paper. Write out a list of affirmations that will bring a feeling of confidence, such as "I am doing well in my English class," "I studied well and know my material," "I enjoy this class." Even if the affirmations aren't believed at first, it sends a positive message to the subconscious which will result in an alteration of the overall belief system, which is the system that creates reality.

If a sensation of panic begins, work with the fear and imagine the very worst! Work through the entire scenario of not passing the test, failing the entire course, and dropping out of school, followed by not getting a job, and pushing a shopping cart through the dark alley where you'll live. This will place things into perspective! Then, practice deep breathing and create a visualization of the opposite situation - achieving an "A" on the exam, passing the entire course, receiving the degree at a graduation ceremony.

On the day of the test, there are many things to be done to ensure the best results, as well as the most calm outlook. The following stages are suggested in order to maximize test-taking potential:

Begin the examination day with a moderate breakfast, and avoid any coffee or beverages with caffeine if the test taker is prone to jitters. Even people who are used to managing caffeine can feel jittery or light-headed when it is taken on a test day. Attempt to do something that is relaxing before the examination begins. As last minute cramming clouds the mastering of overall concepts, it is better to use this time to create a calming outlook. Be certain to arrive at the test location well in advance, in order to provide time to select a location that is away from doors, windows and other distractions, as well as giving enough time to relax before the test begins. Keep away from anxiety generating classmates who will upset the sensation of stability and relaxation that is being attempted before the exam. Should the waiting period before the exam begins cause anxiety, create a self-distraction by reading a light magazine or something else that is relaxing and simple.

During the exam itself, read the entire exam from beginning to end, and find out how much time should be allotted to each individual problem. Once writing the exam, should more time be taken for a problem, it should be abandoned, in order to begin another problem. If there is time at the end, the unfinished problem can always be returned to and completed.

Read the instructions very carefully - twice - so that unpleasant surprises won't follow during or after the exam has ended.

When writing the exam, pretend that the situation is actually simply the completion of homework within a library, or at home. This will assist in forming a relaxed atmosphere, and will allow the brain extra focus for the complex thinking function.

Begin the exam with all of the questions with which the most confidence is felt. This will build the confidence level regarding the entire exam and will begin a quality momentum. This will also create encouragement for trying the problems where uncertainty resides.

Going with the "gut instinct" is always the way to go when solving a problem. Second guessing should be avoided at all costs. Have confidence in the ability to do well.

For essay questions, create an outline in advance that will keep the mind organized and make certain that all of the points are remembered. For multiple choice, read every answer, even if the correct one has been spotted - a better one may exist.

Continue at a pace that is reasonable and not rushed, in order to be able to work carefully. Provide enough time to go over the answers at the end, to check for small errors that can be corrected.

Should a feeling of panic begin, breathe deeply, and think of the feeling of the body releasing sand through its pores. Visualize a calm, peaceful place, and include all of the sights, sounds and sensations of this image. Continue the deep breathing, and take a few minutes to continue this with closed eyes. When all is well again, return to the test.

If a "blanking" occurs for a certain question, skip it and move on to the next question. There will be time to return to the other question later. Get everything done that can be done, first, to guarantee all the grades that can be compiled, and to build all of the confidence possible. Then return to the weaker questions to build the marks from there.

Remember, one's own reality can be created, so as long as the belief is there, success will follow. And remember: anxiety can happen later, right now, there's an exam to be written!

After the examination is complete, whether there is a feeling for a good grade or a bad grade, don't dwell on the exam, and be certain to follow through on the reward that was promised...and enjoy it! Don't dwell on any mistakes that have been made, as there is nothing that can be done at this point anyway.

Additionally, don't begin to study for the next test right away. Do something relaxing for a while, and let the mind relax and prepare itself to begin absorbing information again.

From the results of the exam - both the grade and the entire experience, be certain to learn from what has gone on. Perfect studying habits and work some more on confidence in order to make the next examination experience even better than the last one.

Learn to avoid places where openings occurred for laziness, procrastination and day dreaming.

Use the time between this exam and the next one to better learn to relax, even learning to relax on cue, so that any anxiety can be controlled during the next exam. Learn how to relax the body. Slouch in your chair if that helps. Tighten and then relax all of the different muscle groups, one group at a time, beginning with the feet and then working all the way up to the neck and face. This will ultimately relax the muscles more than they were to begin with. Learn how to breathe deeply and comfortably, and focus on this breathing going in and out as a relaxing thought. With every exhale, repeat the word "relax."

As common as test anxiety is, it is very possible to overcome it. Make yourself one of the test-takers who overcome this frustrating hindrance.

Special Report: Retaking the Test: What Are Your Chances at Improving Your Score?

After going through the experience of taking a major test, many test takers feel that once is enough. The test usually comes during a period of transition in the test taker's life, and taking the test is only one of a series of important events. With so many distractions and conflicting recommendations, it may be difficult for a test taker to rationally determine whether or not he should retake the test after viewing his scores.

The importance of the test usually only adds to the burden of the retake decision. However, don't be swayed by emotion. There a few simple questions that you can ask yourself to guide you as you try to determine whether a retake would improve your score:

1. What went wrong? Why wasn't your score what you expected?

Can you point to a single factor or problem that you feel caused the low score? Were you sick on test day? Was there an emotional upheaval in your life that caused a distraction? Were you late for the test or not able to use the full time allotment? If you can point to any of these specific, individual problems, then a retake should definitely be considered.

2. Is there enough time to improve?

Many problems that may show up in your score report may take a lot of time for improvement. A deficiency in a particular math skill may require weeks or months of tutoring and studying to improve. If you have enough time to improve an identified weakness, then a retake should definitely be considered.

3. How will additional scores be used? Will a score average, highest score, or most recent score be used?

Different test scores may be handled completely differently. If you've taken the test multiple times, sometimes your highest score is used, sometimes your average score is computed and used, and sometimes your most recent score is used. Make sure you understand what method will be used to evaluate your scores, and use that to help you determine whether a retake should be considered.

4. Are my practice test scores significantly higher than my actual test score?

If you have taken a lot of practice tests and are consistently scoring at a much higher level than your actual test score, then you should consider a retake. However, if you've taken five practice tests and only one of your scores was higher than your actual test score, or if your practice test scores were only slightly higher than your actual test score, then it is unlikely that you will significantly increase your score.

5. Do I need perfect scores or will I be able to live with this score? Will this score still allow me to follow my dreams?

What kind of score is acceptable to you? Is your current score "good enough?" Do you have to have a certain score in order to pursue the future of your dreams? If you won't be happy with your current score, and there's no way that you could live with it, then you should consider a retake. However, don't get your hopes up. If you are looking for significant improvement, that may or may not be possible. But if you won't be happy otherwise, it is at least worth the effort.
Remember that there are other considerations. To achieve your dream, it is likely that your grades may also be taken into account. A great test score is usually not the only thing necessary to succeed. Make sure that you aren't overemphasizing the importance of a high test score.

Furthermore, a retake does not always result in a higher score. Some test takers will score lower on a retake, rather than higher. One study shows that one-fourth of test takers will achieve a significant improvement in test score, while one-sixth of test takers will actually show a decrease. While this shows that most test takers will improve, the majority will only improve their scores a little and a retake may not be worth the test taker's effort.

Finally, if a test is taken only once and is considered in the added context of good grades on the part of a test taker, the person reviewing the grades and scores may be tempted to assume that the test taker just had a bad day while taking the test, and may discount the low test score in favor of the high grades. But if the test is retaken and the scores are approximately the same, then the validity of the low scores are only confirmed. Therefore, a retake could actually hurt a test taker by definitely bracketing a test taker's score ability to a limited range.

Special Report: Additional Bonus Material

Due to our efforts to try to keep this book to a manageable length, we've created a link that will give you access to all of your additional bonus material.

Please visit http://www.mometrix.com/bonus948/nuclearmed to access the information.